Wm. G. Justice, DMin, DPhil, DLit

Training Guide
for Visiting the Sick
More Than a Social Call

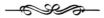
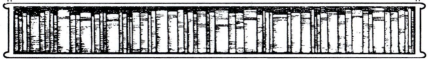

"**P**ractical guides for visiting the sick are few and far between. This author has provided such a guide that is packed full of useful information. More important, the author makes it interesting by including examples and real experiences to illustrate what works and doesn't work in being a caring visitor. He has remained true to fundamental principles of good visitation, such as listening well, maintaining confidentiality, planning visits, and learning from each visit.

Four chapters are outstanding in their practical advice. Chapter 2, 'The Prepared Serve Well,' raises extremely good questions to ask yourself before you visit. Chapters 4 and 5, on 'dos and don'ts,' are comprehensive in teaching what to do (and not to do) in a myriad of circumstances that would challenge any visitor. I found Chapter 8, 'Ministering to Other Difficult Patients,' to be helpful in that it offers useful suggestions on how to deal with difficult patients, such as people who are comatose or have Alzheimer's. Dr. Justice integrates his years of experience into a very readable format that will help anyone who takes visiting the sick seriously."

Paul S. Bay, DMin
Chaplain, Cardiovascular Services,
Clarian Health, Indianapolis, Indiana

The Haworth Pastoral Press®
An Imprint of The Haworth Press, Inc.
New York • London • Oxford

Training Guide
for Visiting the Sick
More Than a Social Call

Also by William G. Justice

Don't Sit on the Bed

Guilt and Forgiveness

Guilt, the Source and the Solution

When Death Comes

When Your Patient Dies

Jesus' Silent Years: Exploring Facts the Gospels Do Not Tell Us

God in the Hands of Angry Sinners

Jesus the Maverick King

The Nature of God As Revealed in Jesus

Training Guide for Visiting the Sick
More Than a Social Call

Wm. G. Justice, DMin, DPhil, DLit

The Haworth Pastoral Press®
An Imprint of The Haworth Press, Inc.
New York • London • Oxford

For more information on this book or to order, visit
http://www.haworthpress.com/store/product.asp?sku=5441

or call 1-800-HAWORTH (800-429-6784) in the United States and Canada
or (607) 722-5857 outside the United States and Canada

or contact orders@HaworthPress.com

Published by

The Haworth Pastoral Press®, an imprint of The Haworth Press, Inc., 10 Alice Street, Binghamton,
NY 13904-1580.

Cover design by Lora Wiggins.

Library of Congress Cataloging-in-Publication Data

Justice, William G.
    Training guide for visiting the sick : more than a social call / Wm. G. Justice.
        p. cm.
    Includes bibliographical references and index.
    ISBN-13: 978-0-7890-2703-0 (hc. : alk. paper)
    ISBN-10: 0-7890-2703-8 (hc. : alk. paper)
    ISBN-13: 978-0-7890-2704-7 (pbk. : alk. paper)
    ISBN-10: 0-7890-2704-6 (pbk. : alk. paper)
    1. Church work with the sick. I. Title.

BV4335.J83 2005
259'.4—dc22

2005002158

To Reverend Doctor Myron C. Madden
and the late Reverend D. Allen Brabham,
my Clinical Pastoral Education Supervisors
during my 1959-1961 Chaplaincy Internship and Residency
in the Department of Pastoral Care
of the Southern Baptist Hospital,
New Orleans, Louisiana

ABOUT THE AUTHOR

William G. Justice, DMin, DPhil, DLit, served for thirty-one years as a bedside hospital chaplain, during which he taught courses for eleven different colleges, universities, and seminaries. He earned the rank of Scholar in the Oxford Society of Scholars, where he subsequently served for sixteen years as Chairperson of the Board of Governors. He has authored more than 200 articles for periodicals, an article on "guilt" in a theological dictionary, and nine books, including *Don't Sit on the Bed: A Handbook for Visiting the Sick; God in the Hands of Angry Sinners;* and *When Death Comes: A Handbook for Pastors and Laypersons Who Minister to the Bereaved.* For three years, he served as Editor of *Chaplaincy Today.* After retiring from hospital ministry in 1990, he conducted private practice as a dually licensed professional counselor and marriage and family therapist, with clinical membership in the American Association for Marriage and Family Therapy. Though retired, he still teaches part-time at Oxford Graduate School and still ministers to the sick through a layperson's ministry program of his local church.

CONTENTS

Foreword

When I began my first unit of Clinical Pastoral Education (CPE) in 1961 at Southern Baptist Hospital in New Orleans, Bill Justice was completing a residency in pastoral care. I learned from him that summer, and I learned from him again recently by reading the present book.

His previous work on this subject, *Don't Sit on the Bed,* has been widely read by both clergy and laity for more than twenty years. I would estimate that at least half of my more than 300 CPE students have read it.

For several decades, Bill served as the senior chaplain at the Baptist Hospital in Knoxville, Tennessee. During those years, he put into practice what he writes about here. He is a prolific author who knows how to express his ideas clearly and concisely.

Readers of this book will be able to approach a hospital with confidence that they will avoid many of the mistakes that hospital visitors make. Pastors will find this book a most useful tool for people on their visitation committee. Thereby, hospital patients will be respected and comforted by their informed visitors.

Richard Dayringer, ThD
Chaplain Supervisor, ACPE

Preface and Acknowledgments

Every church keeps a "sick list." When you visit a sick person, you probably want the visit to be more than a social call. Even if you are a layperson, you want to minister.

During the thirty-one years I spent as a professional hospital chaplain, I conducted approximately 300,000 pastoral conversations with my patients, their families, and friends. That means I conducted conversations with an average of forty persons per day. For many of those years, I was the only chaplain in a hospital with more than 300 beds.

More than forty years ago, while I was still a theological student in seminary, I enrolled in a course titled "Ministering to the Sick." The congregation of the church in which I was ministering then responded positively to a talk I had titled "Hospital Horse Sense." I had presented a simple, commonsense list of things visitors should and should not do when visiting in a general hospital. When some of the people asked what they could read to get more thoughts on the subject, I realized that the small amount of information that had been written about it was gathered from many hundreds of pages from many books.

During the next fifteen years, which included completing an internship and residency program for hospital chaplains, and then while serving as a staff chaplain in a general hospital, I recorded my observations. Visiting daily among my patients, I watched and listened to pastors and lay ministers who truly conducted a worthwhile ministry to their patients. Before they spoke, they seemed to anticipate the patient's possible reaction to their words. They encouraged. They listened. They supported.

However, some said and did "dumb" things that sometimes frightened, discouraged, and even harmed their patients. I listened almost daily to doctors, nurses, and other hospital staff members express irritation about the behavior of family members and friends who visited among their patients. All too often, the criticisms were directed against people who were visiting on behalf of their religious community.

From these positive and negative observations came my first book (Justice, 1973). It remained in print for the next twenty-one years. During that time, hospitals changed, health care changed, and many visiting practices needed to change. As a stamp collector collects stamps, I have continued to collect suggestions for making beneficial visits with the sick.

This book, therefore, is a display of my collection.

After my first book, *Don't Sit On the Bed,* one of the world's most published authors in my profession, the Reverend Doctor Wayne Oates, congratulated me for having the courage to say the obvious. What I say in the pages of this book is not meant to insult the intelligence of the readers. I'm writing from experience, and *I have seen the repeated violation of every suggestion that I will offer.* I will sometimes say the obvious.

Because I have spent thirty-one years of my life visiting at the bedsides of my patients, some of my experience may be of value to you. I think that my experience of training more than 400 gospel ministers in our hospital's CPE program will serve you as I write. I also think that my training of several hundred deacons and other lay ministers in local churches will keep me practical and simple as your teacher.

I am a theologically conservative minister of the Gospel of Jesus Christ. Although I profoundly respect those of other religious faiths and have voluntarily served as a member of the armed forces, willing to fight for the right of others to believe as they choose to believe, I can write only from a Christian perspective. Of approximately 300,000 persons to whom I have ministered in the hospital setting, fewer than 100 were members of the Jewish faith. All others either held no religious preference or in some way identified themselves with the Christian faith. Although I annually attended national conventions of hospital chaplains before I retired, I never met a chaplain from any non-Christian faith. Therefore, when I write, I think in terms of ministry to people who have at least a cultural relationship to Christianity. If you minister through a different community of faith, you still will find virtually every suggestion of this book valuable to those you serve. I invite you to adapt appropriate suggestions to meet their needs.

A training guide is to be read and then used to refresh the mind as the need arises. I would suggest that you read the whole book. Then, before you lay it aside, review all of the material by reading again through the table of contents. While you are gaining experience by visiting the sick, refresh your memory by reviewing the contents before each visit. This may encourage you to read again the details of a suggestion that evades your memory.

I pray that God will richly bless you as you seek to minister to the sick—even to those who may be dying.

Mentioning everyone to whom I am grateful is impossible because the thoughts represented here have their roots in more than forty years of experience. I would have to include my supervisors in training, all the thousands of my patients and their families and friends, and countless physicians, nurses, pastors, and fellow chaplains. I can, at least, name a few.

The Reverend Dan Hix, the Reverend Brad Hood, and the Reverend Phil Groce are all chaplains at the Baptist Hospital of East Tennessee, Knoxville. Dan is the director of the department of pastoral care. Brad is a chaplain and president of the Tennessee Pastoral Care Association. Phil is the hospice chaplain, with many years of experience in that ministry. These men read an early draft of the manuscript and befriended me by offering suggestions that have improved the quality of the end product.

The Reverend Sheryl Wurl, Director, Clinical Pastoral Education (CPE), University of Tennessee Medical Center, Knoxville, generously offered suggestions for making the book more usable for CPE training centers. The Reverend Doctor Richard (Dick) Dayringer, who graciously consented to write the foreword, is a warm acquaintance of our training years. He claims to have retired, but Dick still ministers as a contract CPE supervisor at both the Hillcrest Hospital and the Oklahoma University College of Medicine in Tulsa. With the perspective of a bedside minister, a CPE supervisor, a successful author of several books in our field, an editor of the *American Journal of Pastoral Counseling,* and a book program editor for The Haworth Press, Inc., his words of encouragement as I finalized the manuscript are especially meaningful.

Rita Hodge, with many years of service as a home health social worker; Kathy Sokoloski and Derrance Nichols, workers in an assisted living facility; and Jay Holoback, a professional writer and creator of a lay minister's training program, all gave worthy counsel.

Lynn and Mary Davis, trusted friends, gave creative counsel, and Rick Mays, MD, helped clarify some specific medical issues.

Remaining weaknesses are my responsibility and should not reflect on any of my advisors.

Although the events described in the pages that follow are real, all names are fictitious. Unless otherwise noted, all scripture references are from the King James Translation of the Bible.

As always, when I write, my greatest sense of gratitude is to Ann, my wife, for her patience, humor, love, and encouragement for more than half a century.

Chapter 1

Ministry As a Response
to the Eleventh Commandment

A NEW COMMANDMENT

God needs you. For more than 4,000 years, God has depended on human beings to accomplish much of his work. While the physically ill need a team to minister to their physical needs, they also need a team to minister to their spiritual needs. The words of Jesus provide a motive and a foundation for both.

For more than fourteen centuries, the Jews had lived with the Ten Commandments that God had given through Moses on Mount Sinai. Then, Jesus startled his followers with the statement, "I'm giving you a new commandment. 'As I have loved you Love one another'" (John 13:34). The God of Heaven and Earth, who had given the original Ten Commandments, was issuing an eleventh commandment through the mouth of his son. Jesus did not say this was something he would *like* his followers to do. He did not say this was something they *ought* to do. The King of the Kingdom of God was issuing a royal edict to his subjects—to those who consented to his government: *Love one another.*

When Jesus spoke of "love," he had several words from which to choose. Each of these words has a very different meaning. To speak precisely what he meant, he chose a word translated from the Greek word *agape*. This word is a verb; it calls for action. It has little to do with the warm, affectionate feelings we commonly associate with love. It is a way of behaving. This form of love sacrificially works for the best interests of other people. It encourages. It uplifts. It works to promote growth. It helps.

Those who minister do not have to be "professional" clerics. When Jesus gave the commandment to love, he was speaking to professional people—professional fishermen and at least one professional tax collector. They were not professional speakers, or teachers, or ministers. All care of the sick cannot be left to the "professional" caregivers. Unfortunately, many people view their pastor, priest, or rabbi as having a "cushy job" with little to do but prepare and deliver one or two sermons or spiritually centered messages each week. They believe their spiritual leader may spend two or three hours making those preparations. Then he or she may occasionally visit the sick, bury the dead, and perform a wedding. The clergy are often viewed as the "nonworking" members of the congregation. In truth, most of the clergy I have known work as hard as any people I know. The typical leader of the typical church needs all the help laypeople can give.

Those few members of the clergy who give a monthly accounting of how they have spent their time tend to get the most help from their laypeople. (Most churches have a scheduled time for reports by standing committees and special activities. A "pastor's activity report" can be inserted into this period. Pastors who have done this have told me of the pleasant surprise and appreciation registered by the congregation.)

This report is not for complaining or for boasting. It is simply a method for ministers to make themselves accountable to their people. Too few ministers make such reports, holding to the belief, "I'm accountable only to God."

THE GREAT COMMISSION

All their lives, Jesus' Jewish followers had been taught to love God (Deut. 6:4-9). Jesus had taught them to love one another.

Then, just before he returned to his heavenly home, he directed them to spread the message of God's love for the human race wherever they traveled throughout the world (John 3:16 and Mark 16:15). He wanted it clear that the Heavenly Father wants his people to enjoy an interpersonal love relationship with one another and with him.

Within a few years, his followers inhabited virtually all the known geographic world. Some occasionally made pilgrimages back to Jerusalem, often arriving weary, hungry, and sick. Local believers in Jesus wanted to provide Christian hospitality to their unknown brothers and sisters. They saw a world within their world. They recognized the need for God's love to be made known to the world of the sick. They decided to imitate the good Samaritan (Luke 10:30-37).

By roughly AD 300, hostels were established to meet the needs of the travel-weary Christians who made pilgrimages to Jerusalem. Minimal medical help was available for the blind, the cripples, and the lepers. Some who provided care might have followed in the path of the physician Luke, writer of the third gospel. With little knowledge of the healing arts, and fewer resources, those who served in those early refuges gave the best they had.

Years later, the Christian church established shelters along the routes traveled by the crusaders. Each shelter had a space set apart for care of the sick: an infirmary.

Independent of the hostels, monasteries began to care for the sick and the poor. For the next 1,000 years, virtually all patient care was provided by the priest and the nun. Eventually, when others began to care for the sick, they wanted to study the human body. This required dissecting bodies, to which the church objected violently! Therefore, medicine and religion parted company for the next several centuries.

They began a fresh courtship only in the first half of the twentieth century and entered a tenuous marriage in the last half of that century. Even as late as the 1960s, many physicians still viewed members of the clergy at the bedside somewhat as they would have viewed a witch doctor.

The greatest improvement in the relationship between the clergy and physicians began during World War II. As military physicians and military chaplains served side by side, caring for their combat-wounded patients, many physicians began to notice something that surprised them. Patients with whom the chaplain spent the most time in conversation seemed to heal more rapidly than others.

By the early 1960s, when I served my three years of internship and residency in the field of pastoral care, theological students from the New Orleans Baptist Theological Seminary and medical interns and residents from Tulane University Medical School shared patients and case studies in seminar settings. We also received the same pay and benefits from the hospital (barely enough to survive), and we all learned from the same teachers and from one another.

Members of medical staffs across the country have grown in their recognition of the value of the pastoral care team in meeting the needs of the sick. Several thousand chaplains now serve in hospitals supported by both Christian and governmental bodies.

I've watched both ordained and lay ministers improve the quality of their care. I've watched the working relationship between physicians and clergy improve in hospitals across the United States and in those I've worked in. I have also witnessed the range of ministerial services widen.

Before I retired, I was a member of the Cardiac Rehab Team (for patients recovering from heart attacks and heart surgery), I was on the Gerontology Team (to meet the special needs of patients aged sixty-five and above), and I was a member of the Pain Team (for patients who lived in unrelieved pain for six months or longer). In each of these specialty teams, I was regularly ministering at the bedside and making entries into the patients' medical charts. I also fully participated in case conferences related to each of these programs with physicians, psychiatrists, psychologists, nurses, dietitians, pharmacologists, and social workers.

At the time I retired, chaplains, in cooperation with physicians and nurses in Baptist Hospital of East Tennessee were beginning to join researchers across the United States to examine the role of religion in health. Hundreds of research studies were subsequently conducted, and the findings were published. Among the resulting reports was an article in *Reader's Digest* titled, "Why Doctors Now Believe Faith Heals: Because They're Finding Medical Evidence" (Strohl, 2001). One of the findings reported was that "patients comforted by their faith had three times the chance of being alive six months after open-heart surgery than patients who found no comfort in religion."

Researchers found that people who attend church services weekly are not as likely to need hospitalization as often as those who do not. When these churchgoers did enter the hospital, their stays were shorter. The following observations were also reported: People who attend religious services more than once a week live an average of seven years longer than those who do not. People who worship regularly in their church tend to have lower levels of depression and anxiety than others do. There is also a "significant protective effect against high blood pressure among those who consider religion very important and attend church regularly" (Serocki, 2001).

Taken together, the findings emphasize the impact of your patient's religious faith on his or her physical well-being. Those who support and strengthen the patient's faith provide a spiritual ministry that has a place in the care of the physically ill!

In response to the eleventh commandment, to love, followers of Jesus Christ know they must respond to the Great Commission by taking the good news of God's love into the world of the physically sick. Pastors, priests, and laypeople are practicing an effective ministry. This kind of ministry has been given the umbrella title of "pastoral care."

Whether an ordained minister or a layperson from any of thousands of possible occupations, *you* can provide pastoral care as a member of the health care team. You won't carry a little black bag in your hand or a stethoscope around your neck. You won't carry a tray loaded with pills. Because you have read this far, however, you probably already have what your patients need.

If you are to minister effectively to the sick, you must carry a heart of love, a listening ear, and a message of hope and redemption. You must possess a spirit of compassion, a commitment to faith, and a sensitivity to human suffering. With the skillful application of these qualities, you can minister to the sick and otherwise distressed. With these, you provide pastoral care. With these, you carry good news—the very essence of the gospel—into the world of the sick in obedience to the Eleventh Commandment.

Please do not embrace the attitude that "Instead of providing a ministry to the sick, I'll just pray that God will let the sick person know how much he cares." The truth is that *most people feel that God cares about as much as his people are willing to demonstrate their care!* Across the ages, some of the most significant work that God has accomplished has been through those who work as his servants.

Whether you provide pastoral care as a professional clergyperson or as a layperson of the church, your charge is to quicken the marvelous energies of the Christian faith that influence the body, mind, and spirit of those you visit. Your duty is to promote healing of all that is bruised, fractured, and broken within your patients by infusing them with your contagious faith—your faith in God, the gospel of Jesus Christ, and the soul's endless capacity for growth in the midst of life's most tempestuous storms.

You may even find yourself surprised at the peace many will experience in the course of your ministry. The ancient Jews called this peace *shalom.* It includes harmony with God, with others, and with ourselves. It includes peace in body, mind, and spirit. We seek to promote harmony and all its healing powers as we minister to the sick and otherwise distressed.

The sick are often among those who are the most "otherwise distressed." The issues about which your patients may be distressed may result from their physical illness, or the issues about which they are distressed may have helped *cause* their physical illness.

Regardless of the cause, there are almost always spiritual issues in the hospital setting that need a ministry. Most people are not aware of the spiritual dimensions of their illness and consequently of their need for a spiritual ministry. Patients usually unfold their concerns in the course of a conversation in which they feel free to move in directions of most interest and concern to them. These people, who are ill, are experiencing emotional-spiritual conflict (dis-ease).

A diabetic patient whom I knew casually had been hospitalized once or twice a year for several years because of too much sugar in his system. During relaxed, unthreatened, casual conversation, he spoke of the "craziness" of his behavior. He sometimes drank (chug-a-lugged) a whole bottle of apple juice at one time instead of drinking one small glass as recommended by his physician. He said that drinking the whole bottle seemed to deaden some kind of bad feeling he often experienced.

The next day, when I entered his room, his first words were, "Chaplain, I have done a lot of thinking since we talked yesterday. I think I know what that bad feeling is that I can kill by making myself sick when I drink too much apple juice." I was not at all surprised when he told me, "It's guilt. By making myself sick, I feel that I'm somehow 'paying' for some things I've done." I simply responded, "Sounds as if you would stay a lot healthier if you were to accept God's forgiveness and if you were to forgive yourself."

He asked me to pray for him. I told him that I would, but I thought he should begin by praying for himself. As we bowed our heads, I told him I was going to remain silent for a few moments to give him the opportunity to pray for himself, either silently or aloud. After he had prayed aloud for God to forgive him, I prayed for God to help him to forgive himself.

I saw him periodically for at least ten years. Not once did I ever hear of him having to be readmitted to the hospital with an elevated level of sugar.

For many years, observers in paramedical fields voiced their belief that many patients were ill because of emotional conflicts. "Yes," they said, "physical illness causes us to experience emotional conflicts. But we believe we see evidence that emotional conflicts cause us to become physically ill." During the first twenty years or so of my ministry in hospital chaplaincy, I gave probably more than a hundred lectures in which I set forth the theory that *sick relationships help produce sick bodies, and healthy relationships help produce healthy bodies.*

Others in my field were saying essentially the same thing. Appropriately skeptical, many in the medical field responded with, "Show us. We deal with facts. We deal with scientific knowledge. Although medical science is an imprecise science, it is nonetheless a science. We treat our patients on the basis of knowledge— though limited it may be. Show us hard data."

Then, a highly respected research scientist named Hans Selye appeared on the scene and picked up the gauntlet. His first stress research laboratories were set up in Canada, and others were soon established in the United States. His studies produced what appears to be irrefutable evidence that emotional stress works against the bodies of both humans and animals to cause physical illnesses. Virtually all stress research since that time has been built on his foundations. We can now say that we know that stressful emotions help to produce physical illnesses.

Or do we? Where is truth?

During the first half of the twentieth century, most people believed that peptic ulcers were caused by "stress." Then, someone discovered that it was not stress, but *Helicobacter pylori* bacteria that cause ulcers. (I am reminded of the Apostle Paul's statement that "knowledge . . . shall vanish away" [1 Cor. 13:8]). Now, as I write in the early twenty-first century, researchers are saying, "Wait! Not so fast! We see evidence that suggests that stress at least may be a contributing factor in the onset of peptic ulcers. If stress is not the 'cause' of ulcers, perhaps it works to lower the body's normal resistance to the bacteria that cause ulcers." The jury of researchers may possibly return with a verdict by the time this book is published. If it does, will the decision then go to yet another court? Though truth may not change, knowledge is fickle.

When the truth is finally known, it may be that stress works against the body's immune system, lowering the body's normal defenses, making us vulnerable not only to stomach ulcers but also to many other illnesses.

Many in the health care field believe that at least 70 percent of all hospital beds in the United States are filled with patients who are ill because of emotional stresses. Others push the figure to 90 percent, listing more than one hundred illnesses as subject to an emotional origin. We carry into our physical illnesses the emotional, social, mental, and spiritual dimensions of our lives. Anger, guilt, grief, and a deceitful spirit take their toll on the body. They can raise the blood pressure, agitate the digestive tract, and control our rate of breathing. They can influence the eyes, the muscles of our back, and the flow of chemicals generated by glands scattered throughout the body.

Do not erroneously assume that an illness is imagined because it is called *psychogenic* (having an emotional origin). An emotional origin does not suggest that the illness is unreal or imagined. (The term *psychogenic illness* in recent years has replaced the term *psychosomatic illness.*)

I see evidence that some motion sickness may be triggered by emotional factors. I'm not sure I'll ever again go deep-sea fishing. If I do, however, and you see me at the stern of the boat, green and throwing up what feels like last week's breakfast, do not insult me by suggesting that I am imagining that I am sick. When I'm in that condition, *I am sick!*

Whether your patient's illness has been spawned by emotional conflict or your patient is experiencing emotional conflict because of his or her physical illness is not of particular importance to your ministry. Be assured, however, that your patients are experiencing emotional and spiritual conflicts. They are struggling with them at some level of awareness when you enter their world to minister.

Many people believe that they cannot "minister" unless they have been "called." They feel they cannot volunteer but must be "drafted" into our Lord's service. Indeed, many members of the clergy believe one cannot be a true minister unless he or she is virtually forced to do so by God's Holy Spirit.

Although my call to gospel ministry was personally dramatic, I have reflected much on the call of the prophet Isaiah as described in the book of Isaiah, chapters 5 and 6. Isaiah was worshipping in the temple when he heard the voice of the Lord speaking words of warning concerning his people. God wanted a spokesman—a prophet. God asked, "Whom shall I send?" (Isa. 6: 8).

I envision Isaiah responding like a little first-grade boy, jumping up and down with his hand in the air, yelling, "Here I am. Send me!" Or perhaps he stood in such reverence before the Almighty that he fell flat on his face, unable even to lift his head, but whispered, "Here I am. Send me." When Isaiah volunteered, God gave him an assignment for ministry, and minister he did—as a volunteer.

Before you read any further, if you have not already done so, I would encourage you to pause, lay this book aside, and pray. Offer yourself for service to our Lord. Dedicate yourself to minister to the sick. Ask him to lead your thoughts as you read the instructions in the remainder of this book. Then ask him to lead you while you attempt to serve those who are ill.

Chapter 2

The Prepared Serve Well

PREPARE YOURSELF SPIRITUALLY

You are going to enter the world of the sick. If you have not made the kind of commitment I encouraged you to make at the end of Chapter 1, do so now! If you have not made a fresh, prayerful commitment to serve our Lord by serving others, do so before you visit the next person on your list. "Not my will, but thine be done. Please use me to bring comfort and to promote growth in each person I plan to visit today," is the sort of prayer we make in preparation for ministry to the sick and otherwise distressed. I fully believe this should be the nature of our prayer any time we are about to minister.

PREPARE YOURSELF EMOTIONALLY

When you began dating, your parents may have tried to prepare you for an assault on your passions with sound advice: "Don't wait until you are aroused in the backseat of a car to decide how you are going to behave. Decide first to stay out of the backseat." Such advice is given to young people because we can make decisions in anticipation of an event. Businesspeople call these kinds of decisions "policy"—"If a specific event comes about, here is what we will do. . . ." A similar decision should be part of your preparation before visiting the sick.

Prepare yourself for discomfort to at least three of your five senses. You possibly may see things you find embarrassing. Your patient or a nearby patient may expose intimate parts of the body. The staff simply does not have time to check Mr. Brown every five minutes to see if he has thrown off all his covers again. Mrs. Green may be wearing a nightgown that exposes more than you think appropriate. Another patient may show you a toe that looks as black as a piece of coal, and another may exhibit a wound that is oozing blood—or something worse.

You may encounter odors that turn your stomach. The patient may have used the bedpan three minutes before you arrived, or he or she may have an uncontrolled infection. Another may throw up while you are in the room.

You may hear sounds that disturb you. Your patient or a patient down the hall may be moaning loudly enough to be heard all the way to the end of the corridor. Do not be dissuaded from visiting, but, in the adage of a bygone era, "To be forewarned is to be forearmed."

Decide before you leave home how you are going to react to such offenses to your senses. A negative response can be terribly embarrassing to your patients. It's their world and they are forced to live in it. You get to go home after the visit. You can tolerate it for a short while.

PREPARE BY ANSWERING SOME QUESTIONS OF YOURSELF

As you work hard to prepare yourself, even if you are highly experienced, make sure that you have answered certain questions before you walk out the door to make your visit.

Why Am I Going to Visit This Person?

With the slow evolution of our language, the word *visit,* to most people, has come to mean "to make a social call." If you are only planning a social call, please wait until the patient is out of the hospital. A modern dictionary says that a "visit" is for the purpose of "giving aid, or comfort, or assistance." Therefore, when you visit the sick, you want the visit to be more than a social call. Before you depart, make the decision to visit for the purpose of serving. You probably have no idea of what that service will be. You may feel afraid because you go bearing an empty cup. Later, however, you may walk away feeling rewarded by the Holy Spirit who has given you something to give your patient. Wait and watch and *listen.*

Most of all, prepare to listen.

Do I Really Need to Know What's Wrong with My Patient?

You may not know what is wrong with your patient. This is okay. Unless he or she wants you to know, it is none of your business. If you learn that Mrs. Billings has a bladder infection, what are you going to do about it? Nothing! You are not visiting the patient to provide medical assistance. You are there to minister to her spiritual and emotional needs—to provide pastoral care. You are not there to satisfy your curiosity or to be able to report to the body of your religious fellowship the details of her illness! If you are, you are going for the wrong reason. If your patients want you to know what's wrong with them, they will voluntarily tell you.

Many people resent public announcements in church that tell of their specific health-related illnesses. I've heard patients complain, "I don't want anybody at church to know what's wrong with me. If they find out, they will get up and announce it, no matter how personal it may be."

Of the thousands of patients with whom I have conducted pastoral conversations, I doubt that 10 percent ever told me about their illness. Knowledge of the patient's illness really is not important for the quality of ministry we perform.

Does My Patient Want or Need a Visit?

After all I have said to encourage you to visit the sick, I must also say that not every patient wants or needs a visit. Across the years, I have given many lectures on the "dos and don'ts of visiting the sick." I have most often been challenged when I have said that not everyone who is ill wants or needs a visit. Anyone who fails to understand this statement should answer one simple question: "The last time you had a splitting headache, or you were so nauseated that you felt as if you were throwing up your toenails, did you want someone coming to visit you?"

Hospitalized people often feel too ill to interact with anyone— even their doctors and nurses. I have seen a member of my own family pretend to be sleeping to avoid interacting with visitors. After I had a chunk of my jawbone removed by a dental surgeon while extracting an impacted wisdom tooth, I did not want anyone but my wife around me for the first few days. (I learned later that some people had been offended. Too bad! My true friends want what is best for me.)

When I began the certification process to become a professional hospital chaplain, I was startled when I read the first rule guiding my profession: "Do nothing that will harm your patient." Remember that even if the patient feels up to a visit, the interaction tends to drain the patient's energies—energies needed for recovery.

Doctors and nurses have often observed that their patients worsened between Saturday and Monday and blame this on having too many visitors. Sunday is the day patients get the most social calls. (Note that I did not say that they get the most "visits.") Patients, themselves, have expressed similar concerns. I often hear, "Sometimes, I feel that my friends just wear me out."

All of this is not said to dissuade you from visiting. It is said to encourage you to make sure that you are going to minister—not because someone expects it of you, not because you want to pay a social call, and not because you feel you "ought" to go see the patient.

Do I Daily Communicate Care?

You would prefer not to visit some patients. Their condition or their surroundings disturb you. By their nature, nursing homes are among the least pleasant places to visit. Only after experience is anyone likely to say he or she "enjoys" visiting the residents there.

If you dislike visiting in a nursing home or patients with certain kinds of illnesses, keep it to yourself! The person to whom you make this statement may one day be the patient. We say much in our daily conversations that communicates our attitudes. You may be tempted to say in casual conversation with Mr. King one day, "I really don't want to go visit Mr. Harrison in the nursing home, but I know it is expected of me, so I'm going."

A few weeks later, Mr. King has been admitted to a nursing home. When you visit, Mr. King will remember your negative statement about visiting Mr. Harrison. Mr. King is likely to believe you don't care about him and are only making an obligatory visit. Therefore, he may reject your ministry and even wish you had not come.

Am I Healthy Enough to Visit?

All contagious diseases are not as serious as typhoid fever or bacterial meningitis. To the person who is already ill, however, a common cold may be serious. *Stay away from people who are sick when you are sick!*

My wife was recently hospitalized, struggling to survive a cerebral hemorrhage. When a hospital employee came into her room coughing and sneezing, I felt like throwing him out! I was outraged! If my wife had caught a cold while that ruptured blood vessel in the brain was healing, coughing could easily have caused additional bleeding that would have killed her.

It is bad enough to be ill. Those who are sick should not have to worry about being made sicker by the people who are there to help them—whether employees or visitors.

There's another related issue. If I am hospitalized, my care is costing several hundred dollars per day. I would not want someone making me worse so that I had to stay even one day longer.

You may be wondering if you can do anything in lieu of visiting when you are sick. You may possibly visit by phone. During my hospital chaplaincy, I called patients by phone when I knew I had a cold—especially those who I knew would be expecting my visit.

I remember one man's revealing response when I told him I thought it unwise to visit in his room because I was coming down with a cold. "Chaplain, if you are as sick as your voice sounds like you are, I'm glad you didn't come to my room today. I feel bad enough without you bringing me something else. But if you have time, I would like to talk to you now about some things we were discussing here in my room yesterday." We talked for a while and I prayed for him before we closed our telephone conversation.

PREPARE BY LEARNING

You can learn from each experience in the sickroom. You may be about to make your first visit, or you may have been visiting the sick for years. If you are a layperson, you might be tempted to defer to the "ordained" minister. Most ordained gospel ministers, however, have no more training in visiting the sick than you. They have learned a little at a time—mostly by experience.

Take time to yourself for reflection after each visit. (Every professional hospital chaplain has been required to do this hundreds of times.) With nothing on a sheet of paper that would identify the patient in any way, make notes to yourself as you quietly rethink the visit. Ask yourself, "What did my patient say? Did I respond directly, or did I change the subject? If I did, why did I do so? Was I more interested in what I had to say than in what my patient had to say? (You are not looking for something about your visit to criticize. You are looking for something on which you can improve. The difference is in the spirit of your inquiry.) What might I have said that would have been better than what I said?

If you *really* want to improve the quality of your visits, while you are in that quiet retreat after a visit, write out every word that your patient spoke and every word that you spoke. In a formal training program, these are called "Verbatim Reports." Students who have been reluctant to write one are usually amazed to learn that, after a few reports, they can recall virtually every word of a ten-minute visit. The anticipation of writing such a paper encourages us to listen more carefully to both the patient and ourselves.

Because these reports can be misplaced and viewed by others, make certain that *nothing* on the paper can possibly identify the patient. Your patient will sometimes share things with you that previously have been shared only with God. Therefore, it is not only a written report that you will protect as sacred, but everything that your patient says to you in private.

Almost all of those who learn to write Verbatim Reports do so after they have graduated from a seminary. They usually attend a training center in a hospital with a program of Clinical Pastoral Education. Some study for about three months; I studied for three years. Others stay considerably longer. Of course, formal training helps, but by reading this book you are gaining information that can help you serve effectively. With or without formal training, good listeners make the most effective ministers at the bedside.

PREPARE TO LISTEN

During my years of teaching, I observed that those who seemed to provide the best pastoral care, regardless of where they ministered, were those who were already good listeners or who made themselves good listeners.

We tend to pride ourselves in our ability to talk—to clearly articulate our thoughts. You even might have taken a course in school to help you become a better speaker. You probably have never, however, even seen a course in listening offered. (I taught a course for improving the ability to listen at a local college twice a year for more than twenty years.) We assume that because we can hear sound and have two ears we know how to listen, or might it be as someone jokingly suggested, "Because God gave us two ears and one mouth, he must expect us to listen twice as much as we talk."

In a lecture I once attended, the speaker, a medical doctor, said that he had been taught in medical school that physicians usually hear less than 50 percent of what their patients tell them. To better hear what others tell you, avoid the following situations:

1. Being too hurried—Visit when you have the time to listen to your patient.
2. Having too much on your mind—Clear your mind before you walk into your patient's presence. Focus on understanding what your patient expresses as important. Some factors work against your hearing.
3. Feeling too self-assured—You may believe you already know what patients need to hear before they tell you.
4. Making decisions too quickly—You do not know what people want to say until they have fully expressed themselves.
5. Allowing a personality clash—You don't have to like everybody, and not everybody is going to like you. In the sickroom, however, never argue. Always show respect!
6. Becoming distracted by words or subjects—You may find it easy to become distracted to your own interests by your pa-

tient's words. For example, if a patient speaks of a problem with his mother-in-law and you have problems with yours, you may not hear anything he says after the words "mother-in-law."

7. Lacking faith in the saving work of Christ—Many see our Lord's salvation as relating *only* to some benefit beyond the grave. For many years I have watched our Lord save from discouragement by providing encouragement, from loneliness by reminding of his presence, from guilt by giving forgiveness, and from despair by giving hope.

You don't have to do all the ministering. God's Holy Spirit is always a third person in the patient's room with you. As your patient puts his concerns into words, the Holy Spirit uses you to help make his presence known and to minister through your words and personality. By the bedside, be prepared to hear the most intimate details of people's lives. When facing some of the ultimate issues during a period of illness, people tend to think about their current and past relationships, their successes and failures, and things they have done—both good and bad.

For example, during one evening of visiting patients, you may be told about a mother's death, a daughter's arrest for selling drugs, and infidelity. As a compassionate person, you may hurt as you read the pain in your patients' voices, eyes, and facial expressions.

Beware, however, of trying too quickly to bind up the emotional-spiritual wounds exposed to you. When you see such pain, you probably want to heal what is broken in the patient's world—partly to relieve the patient's suffering and partly to relieve your own. The death, arrest, and infidelity mentioned in the previous paragraph were not from three separate individuals. Each of these experiences were events in one man's life that seem to be unrelated.

This man began our visit by breaking into tears while he told of how his mother had died. As his story unfolded, he went on to tell of his heartbreak over his daughter, who had been arrested for selling drugs. Before the end of the conversation he was wondering if God might have sent these two events as his punishment for his adulterous relationship. It is important to continue listening as your patients speak, or you may never know the extent of their wounds.

During my visit with this man, if I had tried too quickly to comfort him after he told of his mother's death, he might never have revealed his daughter's trouble with the police. If I had tried to encourage him after he told of his daughter's trouble, he probably would never have confessed his sin and his consequent feelings of guilt for his adulterous relationship. My ministry has required that I read many hundreds of reports of pastoral conversations, and I have seen that those who conduct a pastoral ministry too often rush to comfort the wounded. Allow people time to reveal the extent of their distress.

Unless we do, we may be fostering something comparable to the fictitious story of the man who walked into an emergency room with his arms folded across his abdomen. When he lifted his hand, he revealed a small but painful cut that the physician believed to hold little consequence. The physician cleaned what he could see of the wound, applied a small bandage, patted the man on the back, and sent him on his way, still with his arms across his abdomen. On the street, the man moved his arms to his side and his insides fell out. No one had given the man a chance to reveal the extent of his wound. If such a physician would be guilty of malpractice, don't we who minister have a similar responsibility to determine the extent of injury before blindly trying to heal?

People reveal their deepest wounds only when they feel they will not be judged and what they say will be kept in confidence— not relayed to anyone except our Lord when we pray.

A major factor in preparation for ministry to the sick is accomplished with a simple promise—to God, to ourselves, and to others: "That which I hear will not be discussed with anyone beyond those whom I may help in my training." Those involved in the training process must make a similar promise.

PREPARE FOR A TEST

Most people will test us before they will open the door into their lives and allow us in. Some never go to the door when we knock; they are too afraid because someone they trusted hurt them too much. Some open the door and begin their test. Only when they have opened the door and invited us in will they permit us into their "living room."

When you are tested, how will you fare?

The Test

Question 1: Can I Trust You to Keep Quiet
About What I Tell You?

Again, consider the importance of keeping a confidence. People want to know if you will remain silent about the intimate matters they may share with you. I've heard patients say, "I wouldn't tell that man anything! He repeats everything he hears right from the pulpit. When he starts giving examples, I feel like crawling under the pew. I know who he's talking about and half of the people in the church know too." Trust is fragile, sacred, and easily broken. Once broken, it is almost impossible to mend. (Some believe that Humpty-Dumpty originally was named "Trust.")

Medical doctors and nurses are required to take a vow of confidence. The nurse, before God and others, takes the Nightingale Pledge: "I . . . will hold in confidence all personal matters committed to my keeping and all family affairs coming to my knowledge in the practice of my profession." The physician publicly swears the Oath of Hippocrates: "Whatever in connection with my professional practice, or not in connection with it, I may see or hear in the lives of men which ought not to be spoken abroad, I will not divulge, as reckoning that all such should be kept secret."

I believe that every member of the clergy should be required to make a similar pledge as a part of the ordination ceremony. When I have made such a suggestion, I have been reminded that those who minister in the name of God are already bound by an ethic higher than one any human could create. I agree, but I still believe a vow of confidence should be included in every minister's ordination ceremony.

You may wish to lay this book aside for a while and make your own vow of confidence.

If you are worthy of people's trust, tell them that confidences are sacred to you. When someone approaches an intimate subject, you might quietly say, "By the way, anything you say to me will never be repeated. Of course, if you were to tell me you were going to kill someone, or that you had abused a child, I would be morally and legally obligated to report that." (Because laws vary from state to state, you may wish to consult your pastor or a supervisor of CPE in your region for specific guidelines.) When I've made a similar statement, essentially affirming a vow of silence, many have responded, "I have felt that you wouldn't repeat what I tell you, or I would not have told you as much as I have. But thanks, I needed the reassurance, too." Not only does my promise reassure them, but it gives me a fresh promise to keep.

*Question 2: Can I Trust You to Let Me Make
My Own Decisions?*

The sick person may be required to make decisions when he or she feels least able to make them. "My doctor says I need a certain surgical procedure. Should I have it?" "I've heard a lot of bad things about the side effects of a medicine my doctor is recommending. Should I take it?" "My adult daughter wants to move back home. I love her, but I'm not sure it would be good for her—or for me. Should I permit her to move back in?" "I'm not going to be able to take adequate care of myself when I go home. Should I try to find someone to live with me, or should I go to a nursing home?"

When your patients share the urgency to make decisions, they may be needing someone just to listen while they think it through. They know that they often see things more clearly when they hear their own words spoken aloud. When their visitor tries to make decisions for them, they are being told I, too, think you are inadequate to make your own decisions." This attitude is only thinly veiled when it comes out as "I wouldn't think of telling you what to do, but if I were in your situation, I would. . . ." Your patient may be ill, but he or she is not likely to be stupid.

Question 3: Can I Trust You to Withhold Judgment?

While confession is among the great human needs, the need to be accepted is greater. Most of us are so afraid of being rejected that we dare not obey the biblical instruction: "Confess your faults one to another and pray for one another that you may be healed" (James 5:16). One of the strongest fears people have about sharing their faults is being condemned for them. "You might criticize me." "I'm afraid you won't think as highly of me as I want you to," or "Will you still respect me, or will you reject me if you see the faulty me? If you reject me, God probably rejects me too." If we accept people who have done wrong, they are one step closer to concluding, "God really does accept me just as I am."

Your patient also may fear your condemnation of someone he or she loves. A patient who once told me he was struggling to rebuild his relationship with his wife began by saying "Before I can talk freely with you, I need to trust you not to take sides. My wife has hurt me by doing something you probably judge as wrong, but I still love her and I don't want you to criticize her."

Patients you have known before they became ill will remember their estimate of your tendency to criticize or condemn. This means that long before you attempt to minister, you need to destroy critical habits.

Question 4: Can I Trust You to Care?

"Why is my visitor so interested as I bare my soul?" Is it because he or she knows it may help me? Does he or she really care about me and my issues, or does this person listen just to satisfy some perverted, morbid sense of curiosity?" Not all voyeurs are hiding outside bedroom windows, and people know it. Even professional counselors are in danger of becoming professional "Peeping Toms" (or Thomasinas). All of us who listen to others while they bare their souls must not fall to this level. We have to ask ourselves continually, "Am I listening because I may be of value to this person by doing so, or is it to satisfy my own sense of curiosity?"

Be aware that some patients will question, "Does the person who comes to minister care enough to listen to me? Or will he or she interrupt just as I begin to open up and offer a too simple solution to my distress? Will my visitor tell me the same thing others keep saying, 'Just pray about it and everything will work out okay.' Don't I have some part in solving problems I've helped to create?"

Question 5: Can I Trust You to Take Me Seriously?

Most people have at least a few secret fears. They have thoughts, feelings, impulses, or urges that make them feel isolated and different from everybody else. They are afraid that if they reveal some of their secrets they will evoke a laugh or a label of "crazy."

Perhaps a patient wants to tell you about an unexpected "visit" by his father who has been dead for a long time, or his occasional feelings of omnipotence (that his feelings of anger might cause someone to die just because he has a fleeting wish for it), or the halo he sees around certain people. Although all of these experiences are far more common than we think, we are too afraid of other people's reaction to speak about them. We don't want others to laugh at things that seem serious to us. It hurts too much. That which people tell us seriously should be taken seriously.

Question 6: Can I Trust You to Refrain from Trying to Answer Unanswerable Questions?

When patients ask, "Why God?" they will wonder if their visitor will try to convince them that "God knows best" or give them some other answer that ends up blaming God for their sickness. While reading the Bible, I have reminded myself many times that Job's friends served him quite well as long as they sat and listened to his struggles. When they began to talk, they only added to his pain.

Question 7: Can I Trust You to Keep Me Safe?

Before people share important issues, they want to feel sure that they will not be hurt. The quest for a confidant is largely a quest for freedom, and it is often a frightening journey. By unveiling, they put down their defenses and become vulnerable—opening themselves to injury by rejection, scorn, criticism, or condemnation.

The issues the patient talks about may not be fresh. They may be old. They usually evoke fresh pain, however, when they are put into words again.

Women question their safety with a man with whom they might share their deeper thoughts, memories, concerns, or feelings. Men similarly wonder about women with whom they consider sharing their secret side. "If I trust this person with my feelings, will he or she try to take advantage of them? Is he or she trying to seduce me?"

Unveiling one's self emotionally can feel like undressing physically. When emotional nudity parallels physical nudity, erotic feelings can be aroused. Both the speaker and the listener sense it.

When such feelings are permitted to stimulate action, both people are harmed. If you have not already done so, make your decision now, "Under no circumstance will I act inappropriately with the person to whom I should minister."

Let's admit it. Some people seek to exploit others for personal gain. Even clergymen have gained reputations as "womanizers," and more are suspects. All who are courageous enough to tell their deepest concerns have the right to be safe.

Now we have arrived at one of the most important issues of the examination. It's a subquestion to the one with which we are dealing: "Is this man or woman a 'confidence' person or a person worthy of my confidence?" If this is a "confidence man," he is "out for what he can get." If this is someone worthy of confidence, true to his ministry, he seeks to gain people's trust because he is there for what he can give. It is in search for this difference that people examine us. *It simply sounds too good to be true that the reason we struggle to attain people's confidence is to make it possible for us to give to them.*

You might wonder, "When I visit the sick, are people truly inclined to share their deepest concerns with me?" Experience has convinced me that people all around us are eagerly searching for someone who will listen to them. They have something important, to them, that they need to share with someone who cares. I'm not suggesting that everyone has a "problem" about which they feel the need to talk. I suspect, however, that most have concerns they want to share.

As I sit here writing, I cannot think of any special "problem" that I have. If given the opportunity, however, I would probably talk quite freely about my concern for my wife's health, or my concern for our son, whose work requires him to drive and fly thousands of miles each month.

I once believed that people share their deepest concerns with me because I am a minister. Experience has taught me otherwise. They share when they sense that I care.

For instance: I picked up a man who was standing at the side of the road behind a steaming car. He had a small child in his arms. By the time I had driven them five miles, he had told me of his wife's serious illness and his concern that she might die. As he got out of my car at a repair shop, he paused and said, "I don't know who you are, mister, but thanks for listening to me." He had no idea that I was a minister.

Again: I was standing at a cash register returning an undersized shirt that my wife had bought me. When the clerk commented that she didn't have a man to give to any more, I responded, "Sounds as if you may have lost your man." Tears filled her eyes and she spent the next ten minutes, standing there at the cash register, sharing her pain with me. We were strangers. She did not know that I was a minister. I was simply listening to her. From her statement, I drew a conclusion. Then I stated back to her what I thought I had heard her say.

Another: I was demonstrating my skill at the wood-turning lathe during a craft fair in Gatlinburg, Tennessee. I was dressed in jeans, a plaid shirt, an old GI cap, with a bandanna around my neck. I had shavings and wood dust from head to foot. Several people opened up to me one day. One man told me he felt eaten alive by guilt for "shacking up" in a local motel with a girlfriend when his wife thought he was on a business trip. After commenting on my work at the lathe, he admitted he was in town now with a girlfriend. Something in his voice spoke as much as his words. I responded, "You don't sound very happy about being here with her." Ten minutes later he decided he had to go home, straighten out his relationship with God, and give his wife a better husband.

Later that day, a teenaged boy shared his pain after a bitter verbal exchange with his parents only a few minutes earlier. After he volunteered that his mom and dad were pretty angry, I asked something similar to, "Did they have absolutely no reason to be angry?" A little while later, he decided he needed to go back to them and apologize for having caused them to worry when he had failed to call and let them know he was okay at a friend's party.

Another man told me how he had been traveling aimlessly all over the country for more than three months. He was trying to "clear his head" and "find himself" after his wife had died.

None of these people had any way of knowing that I was a minister. To them, I was just another mountaineer demonstrating his craft. Listening is a habit I began developing while I was still a teenager after reading Dale Carnegie's book *How to Win Friends and Influence People* (Carnegie, 1982). With each of the people I just mentioned, I was listening and responding to what I heard.

I'll relate one last experience and then move on. I was filling my tank with gasoline when a man walked up and asked directions to a nearby business establishment. On the seat of my car lay my book *Guilt and Forgiveness* (Justice, 1980). I saw him look at the book, and under his breath he muttered, "Damn! What a load!" I responded, "Sounds like you've got your share of it." We spent the next half hour beside my car as I listened to his confession and pointed him to Christ as the source of the solution for his guilt. As I mentioned earlier, the fewer questions I ask, the more people share with me.

Prepare yourself before you begin to visit by making the decision to listen carefully to what your patients say to you by word, by facial expression, and by tone of voice. Your patients will communicate with all of these. Then respond by speaking to what they have communicated to you. If they begin to cry, you haven't done anything wrong. Instead of apologizing, give them permission to continue. Their tears are fulfilling a need they have.

PREPARE BY LEARNING THE PATIENT'S LIKES AND DISLIKES

I enjoy the fragrances of my wife's perfumes and lotions. I enjoy receiving a bottle of good-smelling aftershave or cologne on Father's Day. I also know that not everyone shares my tastes. Indeed, some are offended or even allergic to some of these things that I enjoy most! Therefore, when I visit the sick, I wear no fragrances, and neither should you.

When people are ill, their likes and dislikes often change. Sensitivities often are heightened. Sounds they usually enjoy disturb them. Foods they usually enjoy, they cannot bear to see or smell. Even if the patient would enjoy them, the doctor may have temporarily removed them from the diet.

I have sometimes suspected that at least half of all the fruit in the beautiful baskets taken to the sick are given to hospital staff, other patients, and other visitors. I must have heard patients say a few hundred times, "Please take a piece of my candy that friends have brought. I can't eat it." Before taking any food to a patient, call the hospital and ask the attending nurse if it is appropriate.

PREPARATION YIELDS PROVEN BENEFITS

Having taught many hundreds of lay ministers in their own churches has convinced me that, with minimal training, laypeople can practice a very worthy, respected, and praiseworthy ministry.

One Sunday morning I was scheduled to preach in the absence of the pastor at a large church in Oak Ridge, Tennessee. In my introductory comments, I remarked that I understood their church had a highly active group of fifty ministering deacons. The congregation burst into an instantaneous, spontaneous applause! I stood stunned. In nearly fifty years in gospel ministry, never before or since have I heard such an arousing response to anything I have said in the pulpit. These people were proud of their lay ministers! They were proud of their laypeople who were practicing pastoral care.

I will tell one more "war story." A pastor shared this one with me. He had been visiting in the home of a parishioner whose husband had died from a heart attack. As they talked, the phone rang. The call was for the pastor, who was told about another parishioner who had been suddenly killed in an auto accident. That family was having a hard time and was asking for him. He felt the woman with whom he was visiting needed him, but now a second grieving parishioner seemed to be in an even greater crisis. He put on his coat and was apologizing for leaving as he paused with his hand on the doorknob. The grieving widow was reassuring him that she understood when she glanced out the window and said, "Oh, Pastor, go ahead. I'll be all right. Here comes my deacon and his wife."

Whatever your title or level of experience, if you are going to minister, you want to do it right. Whether you are an experienced ordained member of the clergy or a beginning novice, you can conduct a worthy ministry.

Although some may think of the "ill" as people who are hospitalized, those who are in the hospital make up only a small part of those who need ministry. Significant changes in health care occurred during the last couple of decades of the twentieth century. For several reasons that I will not discuss here, only the sickest people are now hospitalized. The typical general hospital today is comparable to the intermediate care unit of a few years ago—for patients only a little less ill than those needing to be in the intensive care unit. This means that general hospitals today are large intermediate care facilities.

Upon release from the hospital, patients may go to an assisted care facility, a nursing home, or their own home. Even in their own home, patients may continue to receive home health care services, including limited nursing care, physical therapy, or respiratory therapy. Others remain homebound, perhaps returning to the hospital a few times a week for specialized therapy, through a period of convalescence. If they are homebound for as long as a year, they probably will be forgotten by their church. (I'll return to this issue in a later chapter.) Whether people need the services of a hospital, a nursing home, or an assisted living facility or they are ill but well enough to live at home, they need ministry—they need pastoral care. You can provide it.

Chapter 3

The Hospital Patient's World

The sick usually feel like victims of forces beyond their control. When they enter a hospital, they enter a world totally alien to their normal experience.

AN ANCIENT ALIEN WORLD OF DISTRESS

In 586 BC, the land of Palestine experienced a disaster. The region was overrun by Nebuchadnezzar's powerful Babylonian army, and the city of Jerusalem was under siege. His army broke down the massive stone walls of defense and left Jerusalem in ruins.

Those who survived the slaughter were taken captive and marched hundreds of miles away into Babylon—a strange, peculiar land. The people there were different. Their speech was different. Their clothing was different. Their food was different. Their customs were different. The captives were truly strangers in a strange land. The Babylonians even worshipped differently. The captive people felt that even their God was far away. They wept and longed to return to their homeland. If only they could worship in their temple "back home," they could feel close to God once more.

A MODERN ALIEN WORLD OF DISTRESS

Some patients you visit may feel a true kinship with those ancient Palestinians. They have much in common with those captives.

Physical Distress

Patients often have entered the hospital after an "attack" of some sort: a heart attack, a gallbladder attack, or an attack of pneumonia. Though no one may call your patient's particular illness an "attack" of anything, the end result is the same. A "siege" has occurred, forcing your patient into a strange, foreign land.

The patient may have been carried away, feet first, strapped (in bonds) to a stretcher. Even if he or she volunteered to go, when it is a matter of life or death, is there truly much of a choice?

Like most people who are taken captive, the patient is quickly interrogated. The first interrogation is likely to begin within minutes of arrival at the hospital. Someone comes in with a three- or four-column sheet of paper on which they write the answers to what seems like 543 of the most intimate questions. Within the next three to four hours, at least three or four more people may come in with an identical sheet of paper on which they write the answers to the same 543 questions that were already asked. Each series of questions will have occupied at least thirty minutes. By the time the same questions are asked yet again, the patient will probably feel somewhat irritated or even paranoid.

Patients begin silently to ask questions of their own: "Are all the interrogators going to get together to compare answers?" "Are they trying to determine something about my honesty?" "Are they testing my mental ability to tell the same things again and again?" Or patients may even think to themselves, "Is something wrong with my mind—or is something wrong with them? These people are supposed to be highly educated and intelligent. The first set of questions and answers could have been photocopied and given to everyone else who needs them. Surely no administrator would intentionally tolerate the incompetent waste of time consumed by too many people asking the same questions."

These thoughts may lead from irritation to terror. "Oh no! *I'm questioning the competency of the people who hold my life in their hands!* If they aren't smart enough to photocopy a piece of paper and give it to others who need it, are they smart enough to take care of me?" Although this scenario may at first appear humorous, to the patient in pain and frightened, and to members of the family who are equally frightened, it is not.

Somewhat comparable to captives taken during war, soon after patients arrive in their rooms, they are robbed, not only of their dignity, but of everything of material value in their world. Some hospitals are notorious for their problems of theft from patients. Therefore, patients are advised to keep no more than a few dollars in cash in the room; all other valuable should be placed in the hospital's safe or taken home by the family. After they have given up their watch, rings, and money, someone asks if they have dentures. "Are they going to take my teeth away from me too?" some wonder.

By this time, someone probably has made them take their clothes off. They are left with only a little "hospital gown" that is barely long enough to cover the essentials and with a "back door" that's always open at the wrong time. Someone has well said, "No one maintains dignity in the presence of one's physician." I would add, "And no one maintains a sense of dignity while walking down the hall with a hospital gown gaping open behind." Sooner or later, someone else will smile and call it an "ICU" (I See You) gown.

Those people who travel far outside their homeland immediately notice the difference between their own clothing and that of the people in the foreign land. Where else but the strange world called a general hospital will your patient see people so strangely dressed? Certainly not in the world to which they are accustomed. In the strange new hospital world, some wear a simple, light blue or green costume they call a "scrub suit" composed of pants, slip-over shirt, and sometimes paper shoes. Others wear long white "lab coats," while others wear shorter "lab jackets." Still others wear pastel collarless jackets decorated with hundreds of printed butterflies, birds, teddy bears, flowers, or other things they would not be caught dead wearing in any other place but the hospital.

In this strange land, the people do not wear ornate strings of beads or leis of flowers around their necks. Instead, they wear a "stethoscope," and it really is more than a decorative ornament.

Those taken captive after an attack during war are often tortured. Throughout the patient's captivity, he or she probably will be tormented by testers and therapists. Your patient learns within the first hour that the hospital is a very hostile land. Patients often see no constructive purpose in all that is done to them. Almost every person who comes into their presence inflicts pain.

Many hospital workers announce, without shame, that they intend to draw blood. Then they come back for more. And they keep coming back for more. (I recently heard a patient exclaim only in half-jest, "No wonder they have to give me a blood transfusion! They keep taking blood away from me for tests faster than my body can replace it!")

If your patient's physician has ordered a test of "blood gasses," when the needle is inserted into an artery of the wrist, he or she may for the first time learn the meaning of true pain! It *hurts!*

The torture seems never to end. Even needles inserted to inject medicines that promote healing still hurt. During the course of your patient's hospitalization, it is highly probable that *every opening in his or her body* will be penetrated with something. If no opening happens to be where it is needed, somebody will create one. The chances are high that during the hospital stay, the patient will be further tortured with knives that cut deep into flesh. Of course, the knives are scalpels and the cutting is a surgical procedure, but nonetheless, your patient may feel assaulted.

Some patients will need physical therapy. When he or she enters the physical therapy department, the equipment may be reminiscent of a medieval torture chamber with its wheels, pulleys, and rack. If a stiff shoulder is limited to thirty degrees of movement with little pain, a therapist is going to force it to forty degrees. If it is limited to forty degrees of movement with little pain, the therapist will push it to fifty. Those last ten degrees of motion may feel unbearable!

Hospital employees are not unkind. They intend no harm. Indeed, having lived daily among hospital employees, I am convinced that they are among the most caring, compassionate people I have ever known. I'm calling all of this to your attention to help you better understand the conflict patients are experiencing when you enter their world.

To this point, I have mentioned only the physical discomforts with which your patients are coping while exiled to their strange new land. If you are to understand their plight, you must also grasp their emotional state.

Emotional Distress

People who have experienced both mental anguish and physical pain have insisted to me that the mental suffering is the worse of the two. Hospitalization tends to be a period dominated by anxiety. Patients often feel as if they are dangling over a chasm between a past to which they cannot return and a future that they are ill equipped and reluctant to face. As if suspended in time, patients often feel that the world is passing them by. (This is especially true for those patients who sit at the window, watching people on the street going about their normal activities. These patients experience envy as well as entrapment.)

When you walk in looking healthy, the patient may undergo a fresh discomfort. (You may actually be exhausted after a hard day of work, but you are on your feet and going about life as usual. Pay attention to how often the sick will comment on how good their visitors look.) If the patient were honest, he or she might admit feeling guilty for envying you, or he or she may feel guilty for momentarily envying a spouse or child, who are truly loved. The patient can't help the fleeting thought that may linger no more than a split second, "I wish you were here instead of me" or the secret shame it causes.

All the while, the distant future seems too remote for much attention. Asking questions about the relatively near future arouses all the anxiety most sick people can handle. Patients who have spent much time in church may feel even more guilt when they tell themselves that their faith should be so strong that they would not experience anxiety.

When tests are being performed, anxieties tend to mount. The patient is almost always asking a silent question, "What are they going to find?" Never let your ministry be misled when the patient tells you that he or she has been admitted to the hospital "just for some tests." Health care is largely controlled by managed care institutions and hospital utilization and review committees, and hospital stays cost several hundreds (sometimes thousands) of dollars per day. Not many people go into hospitals for minor, insignificant tests. Tests are conducted because *something is wrong*. I've been told many times, "The anxiety of not knowing what's wrong is worse than knowing—even it it's something bad. Once you know what's wrong, you've got something specific to work on."

Patients who are having surgery are likely to silently ask again, "What are they going to find?" The human mind truly does not fare well with voids. It just doesn't like them. Where a question exists, the mind tends to supply an answer of its own. It may not be correct, but it is an answer. Unfortunately the imagination can come up with ideas that are often far worse than reality. Like a spiral staircase, each answer the imagination provides tends to raise the anxiety level one step higher.

Almost everyone entertains the possibility of cancer when pondering what abnormality "they" will find during surgery. Everybody has heard of someone who has gone to surgery having been told that there was nothing to worry about—all would be well. A few hours later the family was told that cancer had been discovered and was so far advanced that all the surgeons could do was to "sew him up and pray for a miracle." These are the kinds of thoughts and emotions your patient may be experiencing when you arrive.

Experience has convinced me that virtually every person sick enough to enter a hospital is sick enough to think about the possibility of dying. Even those Christians who have no fear of death tend to be frightened of the process through which they must pass before death. Someone told me, "The prospects of death do not frighten me. It's the 'ing' part of dying that frightens me. It's what I may have to go through to get there that stirs my greatest anxieties."

No matter how minor you think the patient's illness to be, he or she probably has thoughts about death lurking in the background. The patient may have only an ingrown toenail, but in his mind he may recall, "Uncle Fred had something wrong with his toe and they had to take it off. Not long after that, the doctors had to take his foot off. A year or so later, he had to go back and have his leg taken off just below the knee. I believe he later had a mid-thigh amputation a few weeks before he died. Wonder if something like that is going to happen to me?"

Your patient may also be silently wondering, "But what if I live? Will I be able to return to work? Will I have to turn my work over to a stronger, or younger, more able person? Will I be able to resume my normal life? Will I return home only to become dependent on the people I want least to depend on?" Older people fear becoming dependent on their children, and young adults fear again becoming dependent on their parents.

Financial Distress

Unless your patient is extremely wealthy or extremely poor, there is the question, "Am I going to be able to pay my hospital and doctor bills?" I've heard many times, only half-jokingly, "If I can't pay my bill when I leave, are they going to keep me here?" The wealthy can afford to pay for their care without placing themselves in financial distress, and the poor are in circumstances that require someone else to pay for their care.

"Free" medical care is not possible in hospitals. Health care employees must be paid. Nurses, housekeepers, telephone operators, office workers, and all other classifications of employees must be paid. Many are not in revenue-producing occupations. Several years ago, in preparation for a meeting of our hospital's trustees, the administrator pulled the records of a "typical" patient and listed all the employees who had served the patient. All of them were paraded through the meeting of trustees. More than fifty employees had served that one "typical" patient. All of those employees were working to support themselves and/or their families. Hence, free medical care is not possible. If for some reason, the hospital "writes off" a portion of a patient's bill, the care is paid for by the hospital's general operating fund. That fund will have been created by money received from other patients who have paid, by private donations (which are scarce), or by some other means.

Even the best hospitalization insurance tends to leave 10 to 25 percent to be paid by the patient or a second insurer. By far, the highest percentage of all patients are haunted by the fear of a severe financial jolt before they leave. Then they return to the fear that they just may never leave—alive.

Other conflicts are experienced by the new mothers and fathers you may visit in the maternity section. Having served as a marriage and family therapist for more than forty years has convinced me that virtually every new child in a home creates a fresh crisis calling for major adjustments. Before the birth, the new parents are wondering if the child will be "normal." They have thought of the hundreds of things that can be wrong with the child at birth. If it is their first child, the new mother may be asking herself, "What on earth am I going to do with this child when I get it home? Do I really know how to be a mother?" If the parents have other children, they are wondering how the other children will adjust to the newcomer. The mother and father have thought not only of the hospital expenses that have been incurred by the mother, but also by the baby.

They probably also are terrified of the long-term costs. Figures announced by the U.S. Department of Agriculture in the early twenty-first century place the cost of rearing a child through age seventeen at over $240,000 (USDA, 1999). This does not include college. Parents also may watch the daily news and secretly ask themselves, "Should we have permitted ourselves to bring another human being into this 'crazy' violent world?"

Family Distress

While stimulating your thoughts concerning the new mother's need for ministry, I have introduced someone else needing a pastoral ministry—the patient's family.

Although the need for ministry to the sick is the primary focus of this book, members of the patient's family also need your ministry. Patients have told me many times that they think their loved ones may be having a worse time than they. I've heard many times, "It bothers me to know how much my wife (or husband, or son, or daughter) is worried about me."

Never neglect the family of your patient. No, they may not be physically ill—but when their loved one is sick, they, too, are experiencing internal conflict. Every person who loves your patient is experiencing conflict. Therefore, we must also remain alert for possible ministry to the patient's friends.

While much of the family's and friend's feelings reflect concern for the patient's physical condition, they are also caused by observing attitudes or behaviors that are not in keeping with what they normally see. A wife may lament, "He just isn't himself since he has been sick. He tends to be more irritable and short-tempered. He is impatient. He is improving, but he seems down. He's just not himself." Simply remember that if he were himself, he wouldn't be in the hospital. Someone may say with a tease or irritation that he is acting like a baby. Most of us tend to regress when we are sick. Do we not recognize this, consciously or unconsciously, when we place the patient under the care of "nurses?" The word *nurse* is also a verb, referring to the giving of nourishment to one who suckles at the breast. It evolved to include taking care of children and then of anyone made helpless or childlike by injury or illness.

We may be tempted to criticize one who becomes childlike during illness. The sick person needs our patience and understanding—not our criticism. All children tend to be self-centered. They have endless wants and almost as many needs. They think of their own needs and interests with little regard to others'. That's just the way children are. Sickness often causes patients to become childlike because it forces them to focus on their own wants and needs. When a man feels as if an elephant is standing on his chest, certain that he is experiencing a heart attack, except for momentary concerns for his family, he focuses on himself. When an appendix is about to rupture and the pain in the lower abdomen draws the victim double into a near fetal position, he or she will become immediately self-centered. When a headache feels as if the head is caught in a steel band and bursting while someone is twisting the screws, the patient will neglect the interests of others.

Children are dependent. Sickness makes people dependent and can even render them helpless—often to a humiliating degree. How can people take care of their most basic bathroom needs when their hands are wrapped in bandages after they have been burned or when an illness paralyzes them, temporarily or permanently? Their humiliation may reveal itself in irritability or outright anger.

Their dependence creates even more inner conflict. Most adults have people who depend on them; when sick, these adults may secretly enjoy depending on others for a change. Being taken care of can make people feel special, and feeling special is akin to feeling loved. If they admit that they enjoy being dependent on their caretakers, they are likely to feel intensely guilty—"I'm an adult. I'm supposed to be independent. I'm supposed to take care of myself. Even if this is forced on me, I shouldn't enjoy it."

During an illness, patients have only limited contact with others, including co-workers, friends, the church, and the community. They are lonely and long to be "back home." I have often wondered if somewhere in our being, loneliness reminds us of times in our lives when we felt cut off from God. Those who practice a spiritual ministry represent those from whom the patient feels most cut off. Ministers certainly represent God, his church, and the community. Their visits say, "We care."

Spiritual Distress

Almost any time we visit the sick person, spiritual issues are likely to be racing through his or her mind. For many, illness is a time for meditation, if not outright bewilderment. They are convinced that their illness somehow fits into a larger scheme. "There must be some 'reason' for my illness."

"Why" just may be the eternal quest. As I discussed earlier, the mind finds little peace with blank spaces. Nature abhors "nothingness" and always tries to fill voids. When the mind seeks an answer, it may create one, a correct one or an incorrect one, just to fill in the blank. Because illness tends to threaten our earthly existence, we look for more theological than intellectual answers.

The question "why" can be a way of backing into an accusation against God. At worst, it asks, "Why did God do this to me?" At best, it asks, "Why did God let this happen?" We usually do not want to know why we are ill. The answer is generally logical, but, if we apply the logic, we might have to accept much of the responsibility for the illness. Though I cannot prove it, I am fully convinced that at least 95 percent of all accidents and illnesses for which God is likely to receive blame can be traced directly to some human behavior. (Perhaps a doctoral candidate will one day research this hypothesis.)

I have listened countless times to patients describe what they have done to destroy their health. A man who smoked for more than thirty years asked me, "Because I believe in God, why did I have to develop cancer in my lungs?" When I worked on the cardiac rehabilitation unit, patients often told me how physically inactive their lives were. They also talked about eating high cholesterol foods and smoking two to three packs of cigarettes per day for years. Many then assumed that their heart disease had a divine origin (a "theogenic illness").

I've listened to people wondering why they had to be injured in an accident. A few minutes later they mention that they consumed only two or three beers before driving.

I suspect that most illness-related "why" questions are asked by people who want to blame someone else for their own troubles. Perhaps some feel grandiose by believing that, of all the billions of people, the Almighty has picked on them.

When God is blamed for human troubles, listen for signs of anger against God. Even though this is the twenty-first century, we continue to struggle with a theological belief that has influenced people of every religious background for thousands of years.

Theologians call this belief the "Deuteronomic Formula." In essence, the Deuteronomic Formula holds that to good people God gives health and wealth, and to bad people he brings sickness and poverty. The Book of Job addresses this issue. Job's friends held this theological position, and their accusations only added to his misery. Job revealed that he became angry toward God during his distress, and millions of others have become angry toward him during theirs. They conclude, "I don't deserve such outrageous treatment!" Not many people in our culture can admit to themselves that they feel anger against God without becoming terribly frightened of him. They need understanding—not condemnation (Justice, 2004).

Encourage such people to express their anger to God in prayer instead of disguising or denying it. Even in marriages, when anger is thinly disguised, the relationship will deteriorate. Only when the couple sits down and dispassionately discusses their differences are they able to become reconciled.

Most people fail to recognize the tremendous faith required for one to confront the authority figure of the universe with their anger. They have learned from a thousand different sources that confronting an authority figure is dangerous because of the human tendency to return anger with anger. Few people trust their employer enough to confront him or her with anger. They fear retaliation! Most people fear retaliation by God. The moment a person says to God, "I trust you enough to express my anger against you and here is why . . . ," he or she has made a step toward understanding and reconciliation.

It is possible that some who don't hid their anger toward God may turn atheistic. When we become absolutely enraged against someone, we have the ability to "write them off" into nonbeing. We can do this with God as well. A person may declare, "As far as I am concerned, from this day forward, God does not exist." Those who make this decision are likely to reveal it by their irritation or outright anger at almost any mention of God. Much professed atheism is simply an expression of anger against God as they perceive him. I've sometimes commented that if I held their perception of God, I might feel angry with him too (Justice, 2004).

Most seem to tuck away their anger against God and secretly list it among their sources of guilt. Remember that guilt needs forgiveness. I hope you know the One who is gracious enough to forgive. When you remind someone of this, you bear good news of "release to the captives" (Luke 4:18). (This "good news" is at the very heart of both the gospel of Christ and rabbinic teachings.)

I have repeatedly mentioned the guilt commonly experienced by sick people. I believe that most people who are sick enough to be forced away from their normal lives feel guilty. If your patient is in a packed, 300-bed hospital, at least 295 of those patients are feeling guilty. The other five are sleeping or in a coma. Okay, maybe I exaggerate. Perhaps only 293 are feeling guilty.

Common causes are being forced to stay away from work, having to leave their responsibilities to others, spending money on health care that could have been spent on family needs, being unable to pray (perhaps being so loaded up with painkillers or other medicines that they can barely carry on an intelligent conversation but expecting themselves to be able to put into words a meaningful prayer to God).

When the mind is fogged by great physical discomfort and emotional turmoil, it is easy to forget that "the Spirit itself maketh intercession for us with groanings which cannot be uttered" (Rom. 8:26). God is with his people, even when they do not *feel* his presence. You probably have heard someone say, "I feel that my prayers don't get any higher than the ceiling." Their prayers don't have to get higher than the ceiling. God is in the room with them. Jesus really did say that he is with us always (Matt. 28:20). You may need to remind your patient of that. As God lives within you, even you represent his presence.

Patients and all of those who care about them and for them need ministry, even though they may not be aware of this. Stay alert to the needs of the institutional staff also. Unfortunately, they may go for years without hearing a word of encouragement and gratitude it from their supervisors.

Family members are anxious too, and they need someone to remind them that God is with them—not only with them, but loving them. They can be strengthened by the representative of God. When you enter the room, you represent God, the worldwide caring community of faith, and your particular community of faith.

Chapter 4

Dos and Don'ts
Before Entering the Patient's Room

A good visit begins before you leave home, and preparation continues after you arrive at the hospital. To ensure that you support what is best for your patient, let's review the "nuts and bolts" of last-minute preparations. We will approach the visit as if you were going to see Mr. Jackson.

Adequate preparation requires that you always follow hospital rules, and it often requires that you ask questions of the patient's caretakers.

PLANNING YOUR VISIT

Flowers May Not Be Appropriate

Before taking or sending flowers, ask if your patient is permitted to have them. Cut flowers in vases of water are breeding grounds for at least six kinds of bacteria harmful to human beings. Any plant form can carry bacteria, pollen, mold, and viruses that would not be harmful to the healthy, but to the sick they can be. Under some conditions, a patient's resistance is so low that even black pepper is barred from the room. (Black pepper comes from an uncooked plant.)

Inquire at the Information Desk

Confirm the whereabouts of each patient before you go to his or her room. Someone told you that Mr. Jackson is in room 402, but he may have been moved. In the hospitals I have served, every day roughly 10 percent of all patients were transferred from one room to another. If you go to the wrong room, you might disturb someone who needs not to be disturbed.

Limit Visitors to Two at a Time

When we are well, we are not likely to notice that interpersonal interaction takes energy. The more people we interact with, the more energy we expend. This is why many hospitals ask for no more than two visitors at a time.

On one occasion, when I approached a patient's door I heard a loud murmur coming from inside. I knocked, and, when the door was opened, I felt the body heat of the visitors. Startled, I stood at the door and counted. Twenty-seven visitors had crowded into a small, two-bed room. The patient's nurse felt like throwing the whole crowd out the fifth floor window! The hospital staff sometimes seems to care more for the patient's welfare than family and "friends."

You and I will make the limit of two visitors per patient.

Obey Visiting Hours

Hospitals establish visiting hours for their patients' benefit— not to irritate potential visitors. People who are ill need rest, and they need to sleep. Most patient care is planned outside of visiting hours, when visitors are "out of the way."

RESPECT THE RULES OF THE HOSPITAL

Read All Signs—Then Obey Them

Let's mentally walk the corridors of the hospital and think about the many signs you are likely to see on or near the door of patients' rooms. They are placed there for the benefit of everyone.

No Visitors

This is the sign you are most likely to see. What part of it is unclear? It means *exactly* what it says. Unfortunately, almost everyone who reads it seems to think, "I am so special. That sign is for everybody but me." It will most likely have been placed on request of the attending physician. The patient or the family, however, may have made the request. Remember that interpersonal interaction tends to drain a patient's energy. The patient or somebody close to the patient has recognized that visitors are likely to drain energy from the patient that the patient needs for the healing process. Another sign may simply request "no visitors at this time."

Do Not Enter

This sign usually tells you that the patient is receiving care that requires total privacy. It may be a treatment. It may be an examination. It may also mean that the patient is bathing.

Isolation

The isolation sign is placed for someone's protection. It may mean that the patient has a relatively mild contagious illness that requires only a facemask to be worn. The illness may, however, be so serious that the walls, ceiling, and floors will be scrubbed down with disinfectants when the patient leaves.

The sign can also be placed to protect the patient from those who come into the room. The patient's resistance to a wide range of infections is low and should not be challenged. However, don't turn and run. This may be the patient who most needs your visit.

In biblical times, people with a serious, contagious disease were required to wear bells on their clothing to warn of their approach. If others came near, they had to cry out, "Unclean! Unclean!" They were cut off—isolated from their community. Patients have told tell me that they felt a kinship to such people. Those in isolation often feel "unclean" or "contaminated." They even may feel embarrassed, and they almost always feel some degree of fear. Imagine the anxiety of the patient whose doctor has said, "Your lungs are in such a bad condition that if you even get a common cold, it probably will kill you."

The patient in isolation is still being seen by the medical staff. They come and go from the patient's room as needed, but take precautions to protect themselves and the patient. You may be able to do the same thing.

If you arrive at your patient's room and find that he or she is in isolation, go directly to the nurse in charge of the patient's care and identify yourself. Say that you wish to visit the patient and need to be instructed on how to do so safely.

You may be told that the only requirement is for you to wear a mask that the hospital will provide. You may be told simply to touch nothing in the room. You may be told to stand a specified distance from the bed, or you may be asked to dress in a paper gown and shoes and to wear a mask and gloves. Whatever you are told, follow the instructions carefully so that both you and your patient will be safe.

Caution: Radioactivity or High-Radioactive Area

Signs about radioactivity give all visitors a warning. Patients with cancer sometimes have radioactive material surgically implanted into their bodies for a specific time and then it is removed. The patient is returned to his or her room during that period.

Imagine that you are the patient. You are *living* in a dangerous area. You know that people are likely to be afraid to come near you. Even staff members who come into your room are keeping track of the time they spend with you. You know that the radioactive material inside you does not know the difference between cancerous and noncancerous body tissue. How much damage is being done to perfectly healthy tissue? All of these issues and more are likely to be going through Mr. Jackson's mind as you approach the door. He needs your ministry.

Don't walk away. Find a nurse and ask what precautions you need to take while visiting. They probably will be quite simple, such as to remain at a specified distance from the patient or stay in the room no longer than ten minutes. Follow instructions and you will be safe.

Fall Precautions

Signs to warn about the possibility of falling take a variety of forms. Hospitals across the United States have not yet established a standard version. One hospital I've visited uses a printed, plastic sign that says, "Fall Precautions." Another uses only a small magnetic hand with a string around a finger to remind the staff of the danger of the patient falling. You might see a simple, hand-printed sign that reminds the staff that when the patient is out of bed he or she needs assistance when walking. Falls remain the most common cause of injury to hospital patients, and this matter is near the top of the list of hospital administrators' concerns.

The NPO (Nothing by Mouth) Sign

The NPO sign has been a source of confusion for the public for decades. Almost no one outside the medical community knows that it stands for *nil per os,* which means Nothing by Mouth. I've never understood why hospitals use it and am glad to say that many have abandoned it. If it is used in the hospital you visit, at least you know what it means. Whether your hospital uses the NPO sign or one that plainly says, Nothing by Mouth, it means the obvious: the patient must take *nothing* by mouth.

Therefore, you will neither take nor give the patient anything to eat or drink—*even if he or she asks for it.*

If there's no sign on the door, what's so bad about giving Mr. Jackson a cool drink of water? That depends entirely on his situation. For example: patients often become nauseated when they awaken after surgery. If the materials thrown up are accidentally drawn into the lungs, the patient is in great danger of pneumonia. To help protect patients, they are instructed to take no food or water for several hours before surgery.

I remember one patient who asked his visiting Pastor for a drink of water about an hour before he was supposed to go to surgery. The visitor gave it to him. When the nurse discovered what had been done, she notified the surgeon, who ordered a twenty-four-hour delay of surgery. The next morning the patient did the same thing again—forcing a second twenty-four-hour delay. The third time he caused a delay, he blamed his pastor for having given him the water. This did not endear the staff to the pastor!

Quite angry, the surgeon warned the patient that he was going to perform the urgently needed surgery the next morning no matter what the patient ate or drank. He would just have to risk the consequences.

Quiet Please!

People who are ill are often far more sensitive to the sounds around them than they are when they are well. Noise is an irritant to them. It probably is the most common complaint of the hospitalized. When you are on a floor occupied by patients, talk quietly.

RESPECT THE PRIVACY OF THE PATIENT

Watch for a Light Burning Above the Door

As you approach the patient's room, look above the door to see if the call light is burning. If it is, the patient has asked for help and expects the next person through the door to be a member of the health care staff. Therefore, it also says to *all* visitors, STAY OUT!

You may smile at the thought of a visitor walking through the door to be met by a full bedpan. I'm not concerned for the feelings of the visitor who is foolish enough to enter the room with the call light burning. He or she deserves whatever embarrassment experienced. I am concerned about the embarrassing situation created for the patient. You can be assured that, as long as you know that person, that bedpan will stand between you and any ministry you might have provided.

Knock Before Entering

When you arrive at the door, you are about to enter your patient's living room *and* bedroom. Common courtesy demands that, even if the door is open, you knock and wait to be invited in. If the door is closed, you may open it no more than a couple of inches so that you can hear the patient's response. Having visited in thousands of patients' rooms, I have never seen one designed to be able to see the patient if the door is opened only one to two inches.

In any person's bedroom, certain courtesies and privacies are in keeping with good taste. Who but the most thoughtless guest would barge into anyone's bedroom without first knocking and being invited to enter? If you are embarrassed while violating this rule, you deserve all the discomfort you experience! Your patient doesn't.

Go Behind Curtains Only with Permission

Any time a curtain has been drawn around the patient's bed, privacy is expected. The patient is usually bathing (yes, even in bed) or receiving a treatment, or someone may have forgotten to open it, which means you may possibly visit.

Although you have been invited into the room, you must wait until you are invited to go behind the curtain. Simply ask, "May I come behind the curtain?" From this moment on, you will be actively watching and listening for conflict. When conflict is revealed, the curtain stands open for ministry.

Awaken Only with Permission

If you approach the door and see that Mr. Jackson appears to be sleeping, you might be tempted to go away without making the visit. You know that pain, an unfamiliar bed, hospital noises, and worry can rob the sick of sleep needed to promote healing. He indeed may need all the sleep he can get, but let the nurse make that decision. Instead of leaving, go to the nurse's station and tell the person with whom you speak that Mr. Jackson in room 402 appears to be sleeping. Should you awaken him? Should you visit later?

You may be surprised to hear, "Is he sleeping again? Would you please go in there and wake him up? He has been sleeping so much today, he probably won't get any sleep tonight."

Chapter 5

Dos and Don'ts While Visiting in the Patient's Room

ENTERING THE ROOM

Look Around for What You Can See

As you walk through the door or step behind the curtain, before you speak, glance around the room to get your first impression. What does Mr. Jackson appear to be doing? What is his expression? What seems to be his spirit? Up? Down? Does he have get well cards? Are they displayed or stacked? Does he have flowers? What does he seem to have been doing in recent minutes? Does he look as if he has been sleeping? Do you see a newspaper that he appears to have been reading? Is he watching television? Perhaps he seems to be doing nothing.

Everybody is doing something! If Mr. Jackson seems to be doing nothing, what does he seem to be doing while he is "doing nothing?" Is he simply staring into space? If so, he is probably ready to quickly move into some serious, intimate conversation. All that you observe will help give you an opening into dialogue without asking questions. Almost everybody who comes into his room asks him questions. Before you open conversation, here are some more tips.

Make Yourself Shockproof

The last time you saw Mr. Jackson, he looked strong and healthy. You feel surprised at how pale he looks. Could he really have lost twenty pounds in just a few days? He looks ten years older than he did last week. He *looks* sick. Don't let him read the surprise in your face! If he does, he will feel worse.

If Mr. Jackson has been in an accident, you may see cuts, bruises, and abrasions. These can leave scars that the patient may be magnifying in his mind—fearful that he will come out looking like the Frankenstein monster. Although some may view facial scars as badges of courage and survival, most people are horrified by the thought of them.

Any sign of distress he sees in your face will be magnified in his mind. His scars will suddenly feel larger and more repulsive. He is likely to view himself through your eyes. We are looking at one of the powers of suggestion. If three people tell you that you look ill, you probably will feel ill by the end of the day. Your facial expressions often speak more loudly than your words. No matter what you see, show no sign of surprise or shock!

GREETING AND INITIATING THE VISIT

Address Your Patient by Appropriate Title

How well do you know Mr. Jackson? If you are acquainted with him, how do you normally address him? If you usually call him by his first name, even if he is considerably older than you, you should continue to use his first name. If you do *not* know him well or he is several years older than you, call him *mister.*

You may view your calling him by his first name as an effort to be friendly even if you are not yet friends. However, there's a good chance that he comes from a background in which senior citizens are shown respect by the way they are addressed. If this describes your patient, he will think you are disrespectful if you call him by his first name. I have witnessed this type of miscommunication on many occasions. Here's one example.

When I was visiting a lady who was a retired professor of a local university, a nurse entered and called her by her first name, Betty. When the nurse had left the room, I asked, "Dr. Howard, how did you feel when the nurse called you by your first name?"

"I didn't like it! I try to tell myself that she can't help her poor breeding. But I really resent it! I'll bet I'm three times her age. I'm due the respect of age, and I'm due the respect of my position as a retired professor! When I was growing up, we were taught the importance of showing respect for the title people had earned, and we were taught that the older the person, the more respect they should be shown. Instead, the older I get, the more people talk down to me. Sometimes, they even talk to me as if I were a child—especially when I'm sick. I've had people who come in here talking baby talk to me. That's insulting to a woman of my age! I never say anything, but I truly feel angry. I encourage a lot of people to call me by my first name, but, then, it's with my permission."

I assure you, hers was not an unusual reaction. I have made similar inquiries on numerous occasions and almost always received a similar response. Perhaps people would be less sensitive to how they are addressed if they were not ill, but you are going to be visiting people who are ill.

If your patient is young, "Hi" is okay. If you are young and your patient is several years older, "Hi" is going to emphasize the age difference, which possibly may serve in his or her mind as a barrier to ministry. Use "Hello" when appropriate.

Speak to Other Patients in the Room

Although you are visiting for the purpose of ministering to Mr. Jackson, at least one other patient may be in the room. Of course, you will guard against proselytizing, but if the curtain is open and you can see the other patient, speak to him or her also.

When we visit in an effort to perform a spiritual ministry, we really do represent God and his community of faith. A simple "Hello" may suffice, but a full engagement in conversation may be more appropriate. You may find an opportunity to minister to him also. Neglect here could be viewed as neglect by the representative of God.

Let the Patient Lead in Shaking Hands

Never, I repeat, *never* take the lead in shaking hands with the patient. If the patient wants to shake hands with you, let him or her initiate it.

Someone may have told you that a car ran over Mr. Jackson's foot. Nobody mentioned that his right shoulder was also dislocated. He could also have damaged his neck, or elbow, or wrist. I would need many pages to write of all the stories I know of patients who have been injured by visitors eager to shake their hands.

For example, a small piece of contaminated steel had flown off a machine, deeply penetrating the inside of my patient's forearm. It became seriously infected and would not heal. After three surgical operations that failed to promote healing, a plastic surgeon grafted his arm to his abdomen. After that had time to heal, the surgeon planned to then disconnect the arm from the abdomen.

A couple of days after the graft, an old friend walked in. Not knowing all that had happened, he grabbed the hand sticking out from under the covers and quickly gave the hand a firm shake. After cries that brought the staff running, the patient was rushed back, once again, for more surgery.

I've walked into a room and shaken hands with several visitors but intentionally neglected to shake hands with the patient. When the patient has mentioned the neglect, I've simply explained my reason. "Because I don't know your illness, I was afraid I might harm you if we shook hands."

If your patient does not offer to shake hands, let your greeting remain only verbal. Older readers will recall that, until recent years, a gentleman was considered to be showing poor breeding and practicing bad manners by offering to shake hands with a lady. If she wanted to shake hands, she would take the lead by offering her hand to the gentleman.

Stop Speaking After You Say "Hello"

Before you say anything else, just say "Hello," or "Hello, Mr. Jackson," or, if the relationship permits, "Hello, Tom." After the "Hello," stop speaking.

"Hello" is always appropriate. Because most people can't stand silence in conversation, leave the burden of silence on them. If they feel like talking, they will begin with something that is on their minds—probably something that is important to them. If your patient says nothing, the silence may tell you that he or she does not feel like talking. That's important!

Allow a moment for your patient to respond and for you to decide what to say next. Use the observations you made as you walked through the door (those I described at the beginning of this chapter).

Mr. Jackson may look as if he is just staring into space or at a spot on the wall when you arrive at his open door. You could follow up with something similar to, "When I came to the door, you looked as if you were in deep thought." I can almost guarantee you that he will share those thoughts with you. If he begins to do so, *listen.*

If he had been watching TV, you might use this: "Looks as if you are passing the time watching TV." If he has been ill for several days, he probably is bored. Respond to whatever he tells you, letting him direct the course of the conversation.

If he had been reading, or a newspaper or book lay close by, comment on that. If he had been sitting, looking out the window, begin with, "You look as if you would like to be out there." Then listen!

Do Not Ask How Your Patient Feels

Immediately upon entering the sickroom, most people ask, "How are you?" or "How are you feeling?" If Mr. Jackson tells you he feels terrible, what can you do about it? If he were truly honest, he might answer, "I have been watching boring TV shows most of the day. I've read the newspaper from front to back. I've spent hours working these silly, 'circle the word' puzzles. I've been trying to sleep a lot—all as a way of keeping my mind off of how I feel. I have done a pretty good job of keeping my mind off of how I feel. Until you asked, I was feeling pretty good. But now that you've asked and I think about it, I feel *awful*. Why did you have to remind me?"

In the United States, we tend to ask, "How are you?" as an alternate to saying "Hello." To the person who is ill, this is a medical question. Every doctor and nurse who comes in asks that question. They can do something about how the patient feels. You are not there to take care of physical concerns. You are there to minister to spiritual and emotional needs. If your patients want you to know how they feel, let them share it without your inquiry.

Never Ask, "What's Wrong with You?"

To ask about what is wrong is to ask another medical question— appropriate only by the medical staff. A large percentage of illnesses are related to the lower digestive system, the breasts, or the reproductive system—all intimate parts of the body. Coming from the visitor, this question has only one motive: to satisfy curiosity. Someone might just tell this inquirer, "Keep your nose out of my business!" If you don't like the word "nosy," try "crude" or "rude."

Follow the Patient's Lead in All Conversations

Patients are bombarded with questions from the first moment they arrive at the hospital. I learned many years ago that, when ministering to the sick, the fewer questions I asked, the more my patients told me. Many patients will be eager to talk. Expect to feel awkward when you begin learning how to talk with your patient. With practice, you will become more and more comfortable.

Use Silence

Consider a "ministry of silence." Your presence alone says "I care." Learn to be comfortable with silence. Some of life's most significant moments are spent in silence with another person. You might comment, "Tom, I get the impression that you don't feel up to talking. If you like, I'll just sit quietly with you for a few minutes." Then relax! You might then watch a few minutes of TV with him if it was on when you came in. Work to overcome your own sense of awkwardness with silence.

MAXIMIZING THE EFFECTS
OF YOUR PHYSICAL PRESENCE

Your Position in the Room

Think About Where You Stand or Sit

Don't force the patient to move. Stand or sit in the patient's line of sight when you converse. If he or she is facing the wall, walk to that side of the bed. Because you are concerned for your patient's comfort, do not force him or her to twist or strain to see you.

Let your patient face you without having to look directly toward a strong light of any kind. Standing before a window through which the sun is shining directly into the room forces the patient to squint into the glare. You probably dislike driving your automobile toward the sun when it is low on the horizon. Some of us can develop a headache by doing so for more than a few minutes. In your car, you can reach for your sunglasses. In the hospital room, the patient probably can't. Standing with a bright bedside lamp at your shoulder can have the same effect as the glaring sun.

Sit Down and Relax

Sit down within the patient's line of sight. To remain standing tells Mr. Jackson that you are in a rush. You may truly be rushed, but you do not want to give that impression. Doing so tells him that other people or other things are more important to you. Repeated glancing at your watch or a clock on the wall gives the same impression. Although you might have only five minutes to visit, when you sit, relax in such a way that implies that you have all day to spend with him. Give him your full attention. A relaxed, attentive, unhurried five minutes will be received as if it were a much longer visit.

Don't Sit on the Bed

Perhaps this is the time to remind you that every culture has an unwritten code of expected behaviors. Part of this code establishes the appropriate amount of distance from its members that others are expected to remain. It's based, in part, on social relationship, according to which some are permitted or even invited to touch or embrace its members and others are not. In the North American culture, we generally expect others to "keep their distance" of about three or more feet.

I used to feel quite uncomfortable around a fairly intimate acquaintance. Every time we got into a serious discussion, I found myself backing away from him because he "invaded my space." I later learned that he had been reared in a Middle Eastern country, where the culturally established distance for conversation is only about twelve inches.

Patients' beds are their "space." Don't invade it. Visitors must stay off the patients' beds.

We must not sit on the bed even when it is empty. I've seen visitors lined up on patient's beds similar to crows on a fence, usually while waiting for a patient to return from surgery. The patient will be returning from a sterile environment. The bed will have been remade with near-sterile sheets. Visitors who then sit on it can leave germs that cause infections and thus additional pain and an extended stay in the hospital. For the same reason, the bed should not be used to park coats and hats.

If the patient is in the bed when you sit on it, not only are you violating the patient's space, but you may also be causing unintentional harm. Perhaps you should not even touch the bed.

On some rare occasion, the patient may invite you to sit on the bed. If this happens, tell him or her that you can do so only with permission from the staff. Go speak to the nurse in charge of your patient. The nurse may tell you that it is perfectly all right.

However, the nurse may tell you that the patient has an infection (about which you did not know) that could harm you. It is also possible that because the patient's resistance is low he or she might pick up something from you.

Physical Interaction with the Patient

Do Nothing for the Patient Without Permission

Patients who were not thinking clearly may have their hands and arms restrained. I know of a patient whose visitor, by the patient's request, loosened his restraining straps. After the visitor left, the patient pulled the needle out of his arm while he was getting a blood transfusion.

I remember another patient who had a test that required him to remain flat of his back for the next twelve hours as a normal protection from a terrible headache. When a visitor came in, the patient foolishly asked the visitor to raise the head of his bed. Predictably, a few minutes after he raised the head of the bed, the patient began to experience a splitting, pounding headache that no medicine would relieve. *That* lasted for nearly twelve hours!

A patient I know fell out of bed and broke her hip after a visitor lowered the bed-rails and failed to raise them before leaving the room.

What should you do if your patient asks for a drink of water—or if he or she asks you to do *anything?* Signs on doors do not cover everything. You could be asked to loosen a restraint or to raise the head of the bed. Or the patient may ask you to bring a pack of cigarettes. These are just a few possibilities. I think I've heard them all.

What can you do to keep from offending him or her? Without giving time for argument and effort to persuade, turn and immediately head for the door. As you leave, without stopping, look back over your shoulder and say, "Before I do that, I need to get permission from your nurse." Go straight to the nurse's station and tell the nurse of the request. (The nurse is responsible for the patient's care in the absence of the physician.) If the nurse tells you it is okay, go ahead and fulfill the patient's request. If the nurse says it should not be done, explain to the patient what the nurse has said.

Keep Hands Off the Equipment

My suggestions about how you should behave may seem self-evident and thus unnecessary, but I have seen visitors violate every one of them. A few days after writing the first draft of this paragraph, a member of my family complained about the visitor who began pushing buttons and turning knobs on her patient's machine because it had begun to beep. The visitor was offended when asked to leave it for a member of the hospital staff to correct.

You are likely to see a wide variety of equipment in your patient's room. Most pieces are highly sophisticated, requiring specialized training for correct use. Keep your hands off the tubes, knobs, and switches! If they need adjusting, leave it for the professionals.

Communication

Whisper Loudly Enough for the Patient to Hear

The typical patient is filled with anxieties, continually wondering, "Is more wrong with me than I know? Am I sicker than I know? Have they discovered something they haven't told me? Am I going to die?" They also know that people in the medical field have not always been completely open with their patients.

If you are present in the room while the patient is sleeping, you may be tempted to whisper. If Mr. Jackson is more alert than you know and hears you whispering, he may wonder, "What are they talking about that they don't want me to know?" If you whisper, whisper loudly enough for him to hear if he is awake.

The Patient in a Coma May Hear You

If Mr. Jackson is in a coma, assume that he can still hear and understand every word you say. I know too many people who have heard things they should never have had to hear while in a coma. Also bear in mind that hearing is usually the last sense we lose before death. Of course, death is not certain for everyone who goes into a coma. I'll return to this subject again in Chapter 8.

Do Not Follow the Doctor, Nurse, or Minister from the Room

Your patient is likely wondering if he knows the truth about his condition. Therefore, if you follow the physician, or nurse, or other visiting minister from the room, the patient has reason to suspect that you are talking about him or her. As noted, the human mind does not like voids. It fills them in with something imaginative, and the "something" is often much worse than reality.

Respect the Patient's Privacy

Offer to Leave the Room During Treatments

When the patient is to receive treatments, always offer to leave the room, even if the staff does not ask you to do so. When the patient is receiving an injection in the hip or bandages must be changed, the need for privacy is obvious.

Offer to Leave the Room When Meals Are Served

It is not unusual for people to lose their appetite while sick. In the hospital, their foods are different from those they usually eat. If they are on a special diet, the food may be relatively tasteless. Food shoved aside until a visitor leaves will be cold and even less appetizing. If your patient pushes his or her food aside, you should take it as a cue to leave.

Most people enjoy dining with others, but they seem uncomfortable when they are eating while others are not. Therefore, if the patient insists that you stay during the meal, you may find it pleasant for yourself and for the patient if you step out and get food for yourself too.

Offer to Leave During Telephone Conversations

Telephone discussions are often quite personal. If the patient needs to make a call or if the patient's phone rings while you are visiting, immediately offer to leave. "Would you like for me to step out while you are on the phone, or would you prefer that I stay?" would be an appropriate question.

MONITORING YOUR MOOD, ATTITUDE, AND CONVERSATION

Choosing Appropriate Emotions and Avoiding Assumptions

You Can Be Cheerful Without Acting the Clown

A warm smile tends to brighten any room, and long, sad-faced, funeral expressions tend to darken any room. You probably learned long ago that your spirit is contagious. You want to uplift the spirits of your patient. It is easy to overdo a good thing and cross the line between being cheerful and acting the clown.

The clergy seems especially vulnerable to this temptation. On numerous occasions, I've been in a patient's room when a normally reserved visitor has walked in and turned on the "clown act." When the visitor turned on the act, the patient turned the visitor off—like an irritating TV commercial! With the clown act, they became phony—which did no good and gained no respect. I've even heard people say after the departure, "He was acting so much out of character. I'm wondering if he's using a drug of some kind."

Tears Aren't Always Bad

Although you want to help lift the spirits of your patient, don't become alarmed if your patient cries. If Mr. Jackson shares his dread of the possibilities of dying and leaving family he loves, he may cry. If he tells you of his sorrow at the death of someone he loves, he may cry. If he shares the source of his guilt, anger, and shame, again, he may cry. Don't panic. If you have not pried, you haven't done anything wrong. Indeed, you may have done something very right. Guilt, anger, grief, and damaged relationships often contribute to illness. Therefore, the flow of tears may help stimulate his inner healing forces.

Beware of False Optimism

Resist the temptation for false optimism. People who are desperate tend to grasp the thinnest straw of hope. You can easily forget that when you represent your community of faith, to many, you represent God. What you say can be perceived as coming straight from God. If you are wrong, they will feel that God has let them down—even lied to them.

I remember the experience of a minister friend. He was about to leave the hospital one evening. As he left his patient's room, wanting to encourage the patient's daughter, he said, "Now don't you worry about your daddy. He's going to be all right." When he got off the elevator the next morning, expecting to visit his very sick patient, the daughter came running and screamed as she beat on his chest, "You told me my daddy was going to be all right! You lied to me! He's dead!"

Refuse to Be Offended or Insulted

Your patient may feel frightened. He is probably uncomfortable—even in pain. Both pain and fear tend to isolate. Both can arouse anger. The sick almost always regress. They are forced into dependence, which most adults resent. They are not themselves. If they were, they would not be ill.

The last time you had a severe toothache, you probably were not pleasant to be around. The physical discomfort, the emotional stress, and the medicines in the patient's system can all bring out attitudes and remarks that seem "out of character." Your patients need your patience and understanding, and they may need your forgiveness. They do not need your rejection, nor do they need you to tell stories of their misbehavior to others. Remember that what you hear from the sick is a matter of confidence to be shared with none but our Lord in prayer or those who may be helped in a training program of which you are a part!

Do Not Be Alarmed by Mental or Spiritual Dullness

You may know your patient as highly intelligent with a deep sense of spiritual devotion. Modern medicines frequently dull mental acuteness, and physical illness frequently pushes people away from God. I heard many times during my youth that everybody turns to God in times of crisis, and I believed it.

By the time I had listened daily for a few years at the bedside, I concluded that for every person who turns toward God at the time of illness, another will turn away from God. Several years ago, while I was doing some research, my statistician at the University of Tennessee called late one night to tell me of an astonishing discovery. While manipulating my data on his computer he had stumbled into something interesting: nearly fifty percent of the people in my study showed evidence of feeling more distant from God during periods of illness than during periods of health.

A few years later, a doctoral candidate read my research and decided to study this issue. His data supported both my observations when listening at the bedside and the conclusions the statistician drew from my research. I can confidently say, therefore, that approximately half of the people you visit feel more distant from God during illness. They tend to think that God is picking on them, that God has abandoned them, that God does not care about them anymore, or that God is punishing them. They may be able to declare with Job, "Though he slay me, yet will I trust Him" (Job 13:15). At the same time, however, they may feel that God is on the other side of the universe.

People with this kind of struggle do not need you to judge their religious faith. They are already doing this. They need you to remind them that feeling distant from God does not mean that God truly is a million miles away. Their feelings do not control God. Their prayers do not have to "get any higher than the ceiling." *God is with them!*

Here is your opportunity to speak as a prophet (one who speaks for Another). You can speak for our Lord. You do not have to declare, "Thus saith the Lord." You can remind them, however, "No matter how far away God seems to be, he is here with you. He promised to be with you always. God's Holy Spirit is in this room right now and is going to stay with you no matter what you feel. He loves you."

If you know it to be true, speak it with authority! If you do not know it to be true, you probably are not quite ready for the type of ministry I am promoting in this book. This does not mean you should not visit the sick, but it means that the quality of your visit will be lacking until you have grown in knowledge, in faith, and in your relationship with our Lord.

Don't Assume Everyone Is Happy to Go Home

People who have been trained to sell, have been warned not to judge other people's wallet by the thickness of their own. I urge you not to judge other people's home by your own.

The hospital can be a very pleasant environment. Despite pain and other discomforts, the patient generally is in a peaceful, protected setting with attentive and often attractive people catering to almost every need. They sleep on clean sheets without having to do the laundry or make up the bed. They are warm in the winter and cool in the summer. Their room is kept orderly and clean. A drink of iced water is a "call light" away, and they don't even have to prepare their own meals. Their meals are served regularly and the hospital has spent thousands of dollars to get the food to the room while it is still warm.

"Home" may be a lonely place where no one cares if they come or go or live or die. They must provide for their own needs. The residence may be physically uncomfortable, and they may not have the energy to keep it in order. There may also be angry or violent people in the building and no one is truly safe. Patients may be happy to be leaving the hospital, but may not be so glad to be going "home."

When your patient speaks of leaving, what do you read in his or her spirit—in the attitude—in the tone of voice—in the expression? If you feel that your patient is reluctant to go home, do not ask a question! Instead, make a quiet, simple observation, such as, "I somehow get the impression that you may not be real happy about going home." Then *listen.* The stage is set for some serious pastoral conversation. You can practice a truly worthy ministry by listening. If your patient denies it, accept his or her word, but keep listening carefully to everything that is said.

Applying Ministry

An Approach to Evangelism

Over the course of more than twenty-five years, I supervised several hundreds of ministers in training for ministry to the sick. (I taught in off-campus programs for eleven different colleges, universities, seminaries, and graduate schools.) My students came from many different Protestant denominations and ranged from no pastoral experience to more than fifty years of experience. I required each student to write word-for-word accounts of the dialogues they had with their patients. The use of a hidden recorder was forbidden and would have been viewed as a most serious violation of ministerial ethics.) Most of my students thought it impossible at the beginning of the course, but, with practice, they soon surprised themselves by their near-total recall. Each minister submitted at least twelve verbatim reports of their conversations for my evaluation and for class discussion.

I soon discovered a practice that remained somewhat consistent among my students over the years. If the patient spoke of some spiritual struggle, the minister could speak endlessly in an effort to persuade to a different position. But by the third time the minister spoke, the subject was being changed or he or she was leaving the room.

If the patient spoke of some strength of faith, the minister typically praised the patient, but by the time the minister spoke the third time, the subject was being changed or he or she was leaving the room.

The ministers seemed comfortable (secure) as long as they were in control of the conversations. They became uncomfortable (insecure) when their patients were dealing with their issues from *their own* background and perspective. Without exception, every minister was surprised when I called the practice to his or her attention.

When you enter your patient's room as a visitor, representing your church or a spiritual ministry, your patient and his or her family instantly know that you hold religious beliefs. Even if he or she has no positive relationship with God or a community of faith, your patient knows something of your belief system. As I have said repeatedly, listen.

You may be surprised at how often your patients will talk about their relationship with God. Listen! This is only one of a thousand subjects they will introduce into conversation. Listen! Then respond to their questions or statements. Both you and your patients may be richly blessed.

Use Scriptures with Discretion

God instilled the writers of scriptures with understanding of every human plight and emotion. The writers knew pain and understood fear. The scriptures still speak to the sad, the lonely, the discouraged, and the guilty. Physicians look at the patient's symptoms and all that they know of the patient's health and write a prescription for medication. Not all patients need the same medicine. I remember a physician who wrote exactly the same prescription and exactly the same treatment for every patient who came to him.

He became a sick joke of the hospital, and eventually was barred from practicing medicine there.

Choose scripture passages as discriminately as a physician should prescribe medicine. Make a list of appropriate passages that speak to specific needs. Then allow them to be the means by which God speaks. Select passages that you think will promote healing to the soul. A frightened person needs God to speak to his or her fears. Lonely people need to hear passages that remind them of our Lord's presence. Each additional source of discomfort needs an application of Holy Writ. Many of your patients need to experience the spiritual therapy available in God's written word. God usually speaks through his written word before He quietly speaks with that "still, small voice" that only the individual can hear.

What NOT to Say

Keep Your Diagnostic Opinions to Yourself

You may have read every page of your worn copy of a home medical advisor. You may regularly read everything that appears in magazines at your local newsstand. The physician, however, with eleven to fourteen years of education beyond high school, really is more qualified than you to diagnose and recommend treatment for the patient.

Repeatedly, I have been surprised at remarks I have heard visitors make to their patients. "Don't take that medicine. I was reading just last week about all the bad things that have been happening to people who take that." Or, "If you take that you are going to become addicted." Or, "If you let them do that surgery, you will never be able to enjoy sex again." Wait until you have completed medical school, a few years of internship, and a few more years of residency before you offer your medical opinions.

Keep Your Horror Stories to Yourself

Almost everyone who faces a hysterectomy, finds a breast tumor, has a mole that might be cancerous, or develops diabetes will be subjected to at least one horror story. Everybody seems to know someone who had something "just like that" who died or who suffered some tragic consequence. Most visitors seem eager to tell about it with enough embellishment to terrify the patient.

Several years ago my mother developed a blood clot in her leg. When she told her physician the frightening stories some "friends" had told her, he responded with obvious anger, "They don't know what they are talking about! I'd like to perform a 'tonguectomy' on every [expletive omitted] one of them!"

Your patient has a vivid imagination that probably is already working overtime. Be merciful. Don't feed it.

Keep Your Troubles to Yourself

Your patients are concerned about their health and the burdens being placed on their families. They are away from home, work, and play. They probably have a thousand other concerns. This is not the time for you to add your troubles to theirs. If you must talk about your own problems, go to a friend or a professional counselor. Don't add stress to someone who is already down.

Beware of Criticism

Few people seem to like foods prepared by hospitals. Nursing units are often understaffed and overworked. Doctors do not always make rounds when they are expected. Your patient may have virtually nothing good to say about the hospital or his or her care. Listen, but do not join the complaints.

You may have heard negative comments from other people about your patient's physician, hospital, or nursing unit. Do not repeat any of these. You will only support the patient's dissatisfaction and may delay the progress of the patient's recovery.

Evidence suggests that the patient's positive or negative attitudes toward medication and caregivers correspond to the rate of recovery. They can trigger the "placebo effect." (The sugar-coated pill and the injection of sterile water that reduce pain are examples of a positive "placebo effect." What we believe is truly powerful.)

Just as you will not support the patient's complaint, you will not support the object of a complaint. Just listen.

Tell Complaints Only to the Administrator

If your patient has a complaint, do not repeat it to others in your community. Spreading complaints against a hospital or a nursing home is like scattering feathers in the wind. Such behavior amounts to gossip. It helps no one. It only harms an institution dedicated to the care of ailing humanity.

During my years as a hospital chaplain, I became acquainted with dozens of hospital and nursing home administrators. Those administrators were all highly concerned about the reputation of their institution in their community. No administrator wants poor quality in any part of a patient's care! If you believe your patient has a legitimate complaint, even if it is long after the fact, take specific information to someone who can take constructive action—the institution's administrator.

No one can do anything with vague, incomplete information. What can the administrator do if you say, "When my patient was in your hospital a few weeks ago, every time he turned on the 'call light' he had to wait at least twenty minutes before getting help." The administrator is likely to feel frustrated, even irritated. From your statement, the administrator knows a problem exists. The institution may have twenty or more nursing units, staffed by three shifts of employees, so what action can the administrator take without information about a specific person?

Instead, report details as soon after the offense as possible. "My patient, Mrs. Helen James, is in room 537. When the evening shift is on duty, she says she always has to wait at least twenty minutes before anyone responds to the 'call light.'"

If you do not hear the complaint until Mrs. James has gone home, go to the administrator at your first opportunity: "My patient, Mrs. Helen James, was in room 537 during the week of March 27 of this year. When the evening shift was on duty, she says she repeatedly had to wait at least twenty minutes for help when she used the 'call light.'" You are not trying to get somebody in trouble. You are trying to help the administrator improve the quality of patient care for others, and you will have protected the reputation of the institution.

ENDING YOUR VISIT

Make Visits Brief

One consistent complaint I heard during the thirty-one years I spent in hospital chaplaincy was: "My visitors don't know when to leave. I love my family and friends, but I wish they wouldn't stay so long." Make your visits short without seeming to be in a hurry. A relaxed visit of ten minutes is generally long enough. Only on rare occasions will you stay longer than fifteen minutes with a hospitalized person.

There is only one reason to stay longer: Your patient is carrying the conversation (doing almost all of the talking) concerning a subject that is important to him or her.

If your patient is in intense pain or is nauseous, a visit of one minute may be too long. When I've entered a room in which the patient is grimacing or grunting in pain with every breath, I've simply stated, "Mr. Jackson, you are having a rough time right now. I'm going to slip out and plan to get back to you sometime soon. I'll remember you when I pray." (We must keep such promises!)

When You Say You Are Going, Go!—Usually

From the moment you say you are going, the patient is anticipating your exit. When we are healthy, we do not notice the little drains on our energies. However, when we are ill, even little things such as the expectation of someone to do something drains precious energies needed for healing. When you have announced your departure, go!—but not always.

If your patient has tears in his or her eyes at the close of your prayer, the door may be opening for you to perform your most valuable ministry. Before turning away, ask no question, but quietly make a statement comparable to, "Mr. Jackson, something very important was stirring deep inside you while we were praying." Then, prepare to relax and listen, and listen, and listen some more. If, however, he says, "Not really," it does not mean you were wrong. It only means that he chooses not to talk about it at this time. Say your good-bye and go.

Promise a Return Visit Only If You Are Sure You Will Return

The words "I'll see you later" as you leave the room tend to be heard as a promised return. Because patients are more sensitive when ill, they will be disappointed or even feel that you have lied if you don't visit again. Even if you intend to return, you should still be cautious: "I'm not sure I will be able, but if I can, I'll visit you again soon."

Wash Your Hands After Each Visit

I feel a bit silly reminding you that hospitals are places occupied by sick people, and hospitals are loaded with contagious viruses and bacteria—some that defy description. I'm not trying to frighten you nor do I want to discourage you from visiting. Even though hospital employees go in and out of patients' rooms every day, their health records show that they are ill only slightly more than the general population. They use precautions to protect themselves. You can do the same. One of the most important things you can do to protect yourself and your family is to wash your hands after each visit you make.

FINAL THOUGHTS

Pray for Your Patient

Prayer is a natural part of many people's lives, and you will pray for your patient. Be judicious, however, about when you do so. Do not use it as a way of getting out of the room, and do not pray just because you think your patient expects you to. Before you pray, ask yourself, "Am I doing this to meet my patient's need or my own?"

I'm not likely to forget the experience of a fellow chaplain. He had asked a keen-minded older women if he might have prayer with her before he left. She responded, "Very well, sir, if you feel it will help you."

Although you may have an excellent relationship with our Lord, you are not always in a spirit for prayer. Here is an extreme example to make the point: It is Saturday afternoon in midautumn. Your favorite college football team is playing, and the kicker is about to try for the winning field goal. A friend who had been watching with you looks at the clock and says, "I've got to run. Could I pray with you before I go?" Would you really want to bow in prayer at that moment?

Do not ask Mr. Jackson, "Would you like to pray with me?" If he is not in the mood for prayer you will have created a dilemma for him. He may feel too embarrassed and too afraid of your judgment to say, "No, thank you. Not right now." Because he feels your judgment more lasting than God's, he will lie and say, "Yes."

For the same reason, do not say, "Let's pray." How many people do you know who would find the courage to say, "Stop. Don't." How can he refuse without fearing your condemnation? He feels manipulated with good reason—you would be manipulating him!

If prayer seems appropriate to you, offer an option: "Would you like me to pray with you now, or would you prefer that I remember you later in my own private prayers?" This leaves the decision up to him, not you.

You may be surprised at how many people will respond, "Oh, thank you. Would you remember me and my family when you pray later?" My patients sometimes have expressed gratitude for respecting them enough to leave the decision up to them.

Jesus cautioned us to refrain from "vain repetition" (Matt. 6:7). Listen to your own prayers. Are you praying from the heart or from a series of memorized phrases? (Of course, there is an advantage in repeating the same phrases: we don't have to think. We can just open our mouths and let the words come out.) Don't tempt God to yawn and say, "Ho hum. Here my servant comes again with the same phrases prayed 500 times before." You do not say the same thing time after time when talking with anyone else who loves you.

How, then, might we pray? We might begin by going back to study afresh the Lord's (model) Prayer. Considering what he said about "vain repetitions," I doubt that he wants us to mindlessly repeat the same words time after time. Encouraging us always to be prayerful, the Apostle Paul said, "Pray without ceasing" (1 Thess. 5:17). He did not say, "Pray without thinking!"

When you pray for a patient, take his or her concerns into account. From the moment your visit began, you will have listened as he or she directed the conversation.

As you then bow your head, quickly review every subject the patient introduced. This will make your prayers fresh and specific to the needs of your patient.

A while ago I visited a couple whose daughter had recently died. She had gone to bed one night, apparently perfectly healthy, and had died in her sleep. I tailored my prayers to their situation. I petitioned God to help them to adjust to the shock of finding their daughter dead in her bed. I asked God to help them cope with their profound sorrow and recurrent anger. I prayed that God would encourage them to accept forgiveness for their feelings of guilt and to help them to forgive themselves. I had warned them that approximately 70 percent of all couples who experience the death of a child will divorce, and I asked God to remind them repeatedly to remain sensitive to the needs of each other.

We want each visit to be a true pastoral ministry, whether we are "professional" pastors or laypeople serving our Lord by compassionately reaching out to others. We can do this through prayer.

For reasons I've never understood, some people tend to raise the volume of their voice when they pray. I've heard visitors in patient's rooms praying loudly enough to be clearly heard a hundred feet away! Of course, they disturb other patients. A physician on our hospital staff walked past a room from which he could hear someone praying quite loudly. He shoved the door open and saw a visitor praying beside a patient's bed. He called out, "Hey, buddy! Pray quietly. God's not deaf!"

Your Best Ministry May Be About to Begin

We will leave Mr. Jackson in the hospital until he recovers. Other patients will recover enough to leave the hospital but not enough to resume normal activity. They will still need others to provide care. Few people are visited after they have been released from the hospital. Many will not even get a phone call from their church. Your most valuable ministry may be ahead as you visit in the home, nursing home, or assisted care facility.

Chapter 6

Shut-Ins: The Church's Abandoned People

NURSING HOME AND ASSISTED LIVING FACILITY PATIENTS

Unlike patients in general hospitals, who tend to receive too many visitors, few residents of nursing homes or assisted care facilities are overvisited. Some of these people go for months without company.

Americans seem to have cultural bias against "placing" a family member into a nursing home. Families often feel that they are failing their loved one or themselves—"Somehow, I should be able to provide adequate care, no matter what the circumstances." Family members sometimes declare, "I will *never* let *my* mother (or father) be placed in a nursing home." Such a promise may be impossible to keep. *The patient's condition can so deteriorate that no family is adequate to provide the needed care!*

Adding to the dilemma, many fear the community's criticism for admitting a loved one into such a facility. Few decisions are filled with more conflict and emotional stress than the decision to place a parent or spouse in a nursing home. Virtually no one voluntarily admits himself or herself. I'm sure it happens occasionally, but I don't remember ever having heard of a patient who has said, "I hate to say it, but I believe it is time for me to admit myself into a nursing home." We don't want to go, and we don't want to "place" our loved ones there. I suspect that almost everyone has heard horror stories about people who are confined to a nursing home.

To many patients and residents, one of their darkest fears has materialized: they have lost their independence. An eighty-year-old person is no more content with losing independence than a thirty-five-year-old. Most people who are admitted to nursing homes and assisted living facilities are discouraged or even depressed for the first several weeks, until they have had a chance to adjust. Some believe they are at the end of the line, waiting to die or that their families will abandon them. Those who have worked all their lives and made mortgage payments for thirty years and are then forced to sell their home are also likely to feel that for the first time they are "homeless." They just aren't living on the street.

After being in an assisted living facility for more than two years, my mother began to talk as if she suspected that she would never again live in her home. When I inquired if she would like for me to sell it for her, she looked horrified as she said, "No, Bill! That would make me a homeless woman! I couldn't bear that!" If circumstances had required the selling of her house, she would have needed the ministry of someone other than her son—perhaps someone such as you.

Although only a few weeks earlier my mother had expressed gratitude for having such a place to live while she was unable to care for herself, she had never fully accepted the facility as her new home. However, many people do.

New residents usually need about two months to adjust to their new home. Most then begin to make friends and acquaintances, to enjoy the different lifestyle, and to live there in inner peace. Many adapt to their new surroundings so well that they fully accept it as their home and look forward to living there for many years.

HOMEBOUND PATIENTS

Mrs. Thomas's Story

Mrs. Thomas sat on the edge of her hospital bed weeping quietly as she told me her story. Her husband had had a stroke a few years ago, when they were in their early seventies. Despite her tears, she smiled as she described how they used to sit and talk for hours before the stroke damaged his ability to clearly pronounce his words. Even she often had trouble understanding his speech.

She began to feel isolated. Their children, who lived out of town, called often, but these cherished calls did not take the place of the many people she had loved and lost. Mrs. Thomas and Jim, her husband, had been active in their church for more than sixty years, having committed their lives to Christ while still in their youth. They had supported the church by regular attendance and by their tithe. They had enjoyed the senior couples Sunday school class, which they had helped organize many years ago. Their whole lives had revolved around their church until Jim's stroke. It had been more than their place of worship. It also filled most of their social needs.

Then Jim died. The class and others of the church rallied around her marvelously until after the funeral, when everyone disappeared. Not even her pastor visited to give her an opportunity to verbally express some of her grief.

A couple of weeks after Jim's death, when some of the shock had worn off, Mrs. Thomas plunged into a downward spiral of sadness. She feared that she was going crazy. No one was there to tell her that she was experiencing a normal, typical part of grief. She felt that everybody had forgotten Jim because no one spoke his name any more. The house seemed larger and emptier now that Jim was gone, so she looked for excuses to leave it. In the Sunday school class and at other functions that she and Jim had formerly attended, she quietly wondered, however, if she were out of place there too because she was no longer part of a couple. But she loved her church and her friends there and remained quite active.

Then it happened. She collapsed on her way to her car one Sunday morning after the worship service. She was rushed to the hospital, where she was confined for more than three weeks. "When I was so sick that I could barely hold my head up, feeling least like having visitors, I think half the people of my church visited me. The longer I stayed in the hospital, the fewer the people who came. By the time I felt like enjoying visitors, almost nobody came. Then I went home." She started to cry again. "I was too ill to go back to church or to do much of anything away from home." She was placed on the homebound list at her church. "A few people came to see me at first. Then, for the next few months, one or two came occasionally. Now that I have been out of church for close to a year, nobody comes. Where are they? I thought they were my friends!"

She sobbed. Not only had she lost her husband, she had lost her church! My mind flashed to the lamentation of the psalmist who looked about and concluded, "no one cares a bit about what happens to me" (Ps. 142:4 NIV).

I wish hers were a unique story. While serving as a hospital chaplain, however, I heard so many similar stories that I've concluded: *Any member of a church who is away from public worship for a year or longer is abandoned.* There may be a few exceptions, but not many.

Meeting the Spiritual Needs of Nursing Home Residents

If you believe this conclusion is too harsh, do some research. Begin with your own church. Then, call your nearest nursing home and ask a question of the activities director: "What are the local churches doing to meet the spiritual needs of those who now reside in your facility?" Having heard so many stories similar to Mrs. Thomas's, several years ago I decided to study the needs for ministry in the nursing homes of my region. With the help of a local pastor, we interviewed the administrators, activities directors, and residents of twenty-seven nursing homes.

We could have stopped after the first interview. We learned almost nothing new in the remaining twenty-six nursing homes. As soon as we began asking our questions, we found almost instant anger against pastors and local churches. Everywhere we went we heard that, with almost no exception, *within a few weeks of admission, no representatives from local churches visited their patients.* Were it not for the families' visits, their patients would have been totally abandoned. Few families truly abandon their loved ones who have entered a nursing home or assisted living facility.

However, in our mobile society, very loving and caring family members often live hundreds of miles away. No one would expect a son or daughter who lives in Oregon to frequently visit an ailing parent who lives in North Carolina. Under such conditions, the church family has an even greater responsibility and opportunity to express support and love.

Unfortunately, we found that the staff often had to call several churches before finding someone who would visit a specific person whom they believed needed a spiritual ministry. They also had difficulty finding someone to come in and conduct worship services.

We often encountered open cynicism in comments comparable to, "Churches know they aren't going to add any new members from here." Even scheduled worship services were cancelled without notice. No one who has read the published report has come forth to challenge it (Justice, 1991). As an experienced researcher, I know that our ten-year-old study in one geographic region does not speak for all regions of the United States. However, from more recent statements I have heard from other chaplains and nursing home staff members, I suspect that we are viewing a widespread issue. Might it speak for your geographic region? As I suggested earlier, if you dare to investigate, try to prove that our study does not speak for your community, town, or city.

You may believe, as others do, that North Americans have developed a cultural dislike for visitors. I'm not convinced. I've drawn some conclusions based on thousands of hours at the bedside. We tend to dislike visitors who come to get something. Earlier, I menteioned that the word *visit* suggests more than a social call. When we visit those too ill to worship with their congregation, we go to give comfort and help. When we visit the sick, we go, not to *get* something, but to *give* something of ourselves. Those who give are usually welcome.

Those who are homebound or confined to an assisted living facility or nursing home are separated from their community and from their church. You represent both. As a member of both communities, you help eliminate the patient's sense of isolation—of detachment—of alienation.

Your personal interaction with patients keeps them feeling involved, thereby boosting their perception of purpose and meaning. Because you are a member of the church, patients maintain a connection with the spiritual community too. Of all the people I have known who visit the sick, I have heard them say hundreds of times that they receive more in visiting the sick than they give. Is it ironic that in giving of ourselves, we receive more than we give? Although our Lord has said that it is more blessed to give than to receive, someone must be willing to receive before someone can give. Although receiving must not be your motive, if you give of your time and effort in visiting the shut-ins of your church, you will receive a blessing beyond words. Before beginning spiritual ministry to the shut-ins of your church, let's consider the following points.

Wait! Have you read the previous five chapters? I envision someone picking up this book and looking at the chapter headings and thinking, "Because I am not going to be visiting in the hospital, I do not need to read those first five chapters." At least 90 percent of everything I have said up to this point needs to be applied when visiting all who are sick—no matter where you visit them.

PLANNING THE TIME AND LENGTH OF YOUR VISIT

Some patients who are well enough to go home from the hospital may still be far from returning to normal activities. They are homebound. Some people are homebound for only a few days, but others may be homebound for years. Many are lonely; most are discouraged. All are in danger of being abandoned by their church. Only people such as you can keep that from happening. If your church does not have an organized program for regularly ministering to the homebound, seriously consider establishing one. The program I helped build in our church has more than forty volunteer members who visit faithfully. We want to make certain that no homebound person (including those in nursing homes and assisted living facilities) goes for more than a month without at least one visit. We want all members to realize that they are an important part our Lord's church.

Make an Appointment

You might think, "They're not going anywhere. What's the point in calling ahead?"

No matter where people live, in most circles, the day of the welcomed "drop in anytime" visit has gone. When guests are coming into the home, most folks want things in order. They don't want yesterday's newspaper lying on the sofa, or a cold cup of coffee still on the table, or unopened mail piled on the kitchen counter. This condition may be quite acceptable for the family, but when company comes people want everything orderly. If the company is coming from their church, they may feel even more concerned that everything appears tidy.

People also want to look "presentable." Not many women would genuinely welcome an unexpected guest when they have just finished shampooing their hair. A man who is the caretaker of a sick wife may not appreciate a visit from a representative of his church when he has just come in sweaty after mowing the lawn or when he has just stepped out of the shower. You may also hear those who are too ill, too weak, or too disabled to care for the home as they would prefer apologize for the dust and disorder.

It is also important that we call before visiting. Ask them the time of day or evening that they prefer you to visit for no more than half an hour.

Patients always receive meals and baths in the morning. Trips to doctors' offices, hospitals, or treatment centers are scheduled throughout the day. Some patients need a nap shortly after their noonday meal. Exercise periods may be conducted at almost any time. Many people also retire early in the evening.

In assisted living homes, residents are encouraged to take part in outside activities. They may go for a sightseeing drive or to an opera performance. They may be taken for a shopping spree, a hair appointment, or any number of planned activities.

I've heard people who visit complain about "those rude people who kept watching TV while I was visiting." That issue has another side. The person visited probably has a complaint also. If the visitor had called ahead, he or she might have been told of a more appropriate time at which a visit would be appreciated. Many people have favorite TV shows. For instance, when the sick person's college alma mater football team is playing on Saturday afternoon, visitors who want to chat are not usually welcome.

If the patient watches TV while you are visiting, remember that not all communication is accomplished with words. We also communicate with our behavior! If patients watch TV instead of conversing with you, they may be telling you that they do not want to talk. Only if you have coordinated your visit with the patient's desires may you politely ask permission to turn off the TV.

Remember that the unexpected visitor may intrude into other plans. When my wife was recovering from a near-fatal cerebral hemorrhage, she did not feel up to social interaction outside our immediate family. After a few weeks, she was getting "cabin fever" and wanted to go for a ride in the country. If an unexpected visitor had arrived as we were about to leave, both of us would have been irritated.

Another reason to call before visiting is that people are not always in the mood for visitors. Recently, my wife and I were planning to visit a shut-in from our church. When I called ahead, the woman thanked me for calling and said that she had a cold with a fever and would appreciate a visit in about a week. We waited a week and called again. That time, the lady seemed eager for us to visit. We came away feeling it had been time well spent.

Allot About Half an Hour for Your Typical Visit

Instead of the five- to fifteen-minute visit that is appropriate for the hospitalized patient, you should spend more time when visiting in the nursing home or assisted living facility. These patients tend to have too much unoccupied time on their hands. Less than a thirty-minute visit may be viewed as only a token, obligatory visit. You will quickly recognize that some patients who are feeling well would welcome an "all-day" chat. Some can talk for hours. If experience tells you that your patient is one of these, you may need to state early in your visit, "I have some business to attend to, so I will be unable to visit more than half an hour today." You can also make it clear when you call to make the appointment that you can stay for no more than half an hour.

STRUCTURING YOUR VISIT AND MAKING THE MOST OF YOUR TIME

Consider Taking Communion/Eucharist/Lord's Supper

No activity of the church more fully signifies that one is a part of a body of believers than the communion service. After months away from their church, the privilege of participating in the communion service helps to reassure patients that they are still a part of the church. I have seen patients openly weep with joy when a member of their church has entered and announced that they have brought an opportunity for communion.

If your church approves, consider offering it to your shut-ins within the next week after it has been observed by your congregation. From your religious supply or bookstore, you can purchase a small kit for carrying the bread, wine, and cup. Perhaps your church would purchase one to be used by everyone who visits shut-ins. Of course, because the bread and wine are food, before you take communion to your patient, you must get approval from the patient's caretaker.

Eat with Your Patient If Invited

Assisted living facilities usually provide meals in a common dining room—similar to a restaurant. Some even provide a menu from which residents may order. If your patient invites you to eat with him or her, check with the staff. They may be glad to have you as company for their resident during the meal. Because it gives them a chance to "show off" the quality of food provided for their residents, the staff may provide your meal without charge. If they do charge you, the fee will usually be quite reasonable.

Long ago, I recognized that we of the church often experience more communion over a quiet, relaxed meal together than we do in the communion service of our local church. Quiet conversation over a meal can serve as a true ministry—a ministry that may be obvious to the visited, but unnoticed by the visitor.

Keep Your Patient Informed

Although everyone works to help the residents feel that they are in a new home, they still want to maintain ties with the former community. Help your patient stay connected by sharing current news from the community. If a new house is being built down the street from where your patient formerly lived, tell her. If a grandson's high school has won a regional championship, tell her. If her next door neighbor has fallen and broken a hip, tell her. If people have asked about her welfare, tell her. If her beautician has told you that she is praying for your patient, tell her that too. Keep her informed.

Be Patient with Mental Deficiencies

If your patient seems to be experiencing mental deterioration (dementia), don't become alarmed. It may be her reaction to medicines, or she may have some other problem that can be treated with highly positive results. I heard a gerontologist say that, among the elderly, 90 percent of all mental problems that were once considered irreversible are now successfully treated by medicines and/or diet. (A gerontologist, sometimes called a geriatrician, is a medical doctor who has specialized training for service to patients age sixty-five years or above.) As a chaplain in our hospital's geriatric unit I have seen patients' mental abilities "miraculously" improve within a couple of weeks with only a change of diet. (A geriatric unit provides care and treatment of problems most common to patients age sixty-five and above.) Of course, that which works for some patients does not work for all.

When the mind is not functioning well, people may clearly remember things that happened seventy-five years ago but not something that happened ten minutes ago. They may flush their eyeglasses or dentures down the commode and insist that a member of the nursing staff has stolen them. They may have finished eating a full meal five minutes before you came in and swear that no one has given them anything to eat in the past three days. Perhaps the pastor may have walked out as you were coming in and the patient may insist the pastor hasn't visited in months.

Sanitation is often discarded and modesty may disappear. Both men and women in this state may freely expose themselves to you. Once-inhibited words and actions may flow from the patient's lips in language that might be embarrassing—often to the embarrassment and sometimes anger of the family.

Help with Small Errands

What can your patients not do for themselves?

Can they read? If not, you might read them the newspaper, or get well cards, or letters. Can they write? They might need you to write a letter. If they do not have full use of their hands, or have difficulty with coordination, they may need help eating. Do they need someone to go shopping for them?

Patients may feel too proud to ask for help, but would accept it if someone volunteered. If they do not ask you to do something specific, listen. They may tell you of their greatest needs by telling you what they can't do any more.

UNDERSTANDING AND RESPECTING
THE STAFF'S CONCERNS AND REQUESTS

Rules for patients and visitors may seem foolish and unreasonable to you. Many years ago, my son was grumbling about a "dumb" rule that irritated him. After a few moments of reflection, he wisely mused, "Dad, do you think maybe somebody has done something 'dumb' that has forced them to make that kind of rule?" I suspect he was correct.

Though we may not understand the reasoning behind them, most rules made by health care institutions are designed for the benefit of their patients and staff. The institution's staff does not want to offend you. They have more to do than to sit around figuring out how to annoy guests. Even if the staff had no humanitarian concerns, they would need the goodwill of the public. Their public image is vital to the financial stability of their institution.

While preparing this material, I interviewed several administrators and directors of nursing homes. Here are their most common complaints about their visitors:

"They give cigarettes to patients whom the doctor has ordered not to smoke."

"They ignore signs, such as, 'Don't Use This Door.' Then unattended patients can wander out and get themselves hurt."

"They bring candy to diabetic patients."

"They let the bedrails down and don't put them back up before they leave."

"They take restraints off patients who have a history of climbing over the bedrails. We don't use restraints unless we have to. We don't want our patients to fall!"

Give Patient's Medicines Only to the Staff

You may want to do a good deed by saving someone at home a trip to the nursing home. If *anyone* asks you to take medicines to your patient, give the medicine only to the staff. Medical information and patients' situations change daily. A drug that was beneficial yesterday may be harmful today. A patient may also be harmed by taking something from you that the staff already has given.

Take Only Foods Approved by the Staff

Patient meals are planned by professional dietitians who work closely with the physicians. Dietary guidelines can change from day to day. An attractive, innocent looking fruit basket may have been an ideal gift last week. Patients who now must drastically reduce the amount of potassium in their diet are at risk of high blood pressure or stroke if they eat a banana from a gift basket. Therefore, it is wise to ask for advice from the patient's nurse before bringing foods. Then tell the nursing staff what you have brought before giving it to the patient. Also, keep in mind that food brought to the patient creates a storage problem and can be quite messy.

Make Gifts Practical

If you were living away from your home, in a place that might become permanent, what would you need? Try to put yourself in your patient's situation. Might you need toothpaste? Washcloths? Towels? Grooming articles? Lotions? Safety razor? Reading material appropriate to your particular interests? A subscription to a favorite magazine keeps giving for a year. Would you need underwear? Pajamas or gown? (All clothing should be labeled with the owner's name to help keep it from getting misplaced in the institution's laundry.) The patient probably needs stamps, envelopes, a pen or pencil, and stationary. These are appreciated even by patients who need someone to write for them. How about notecards and postcards? When you think of something that might be appropriate, ask the patient or staff.

In their excellent book, *A Guide to Nursing Home Living,* Jerry Griffith and Twila Standberg offer excellent gift suggestions. Because spices can bring back fond memories of favorite places and people, the authors suggest making a spice bottle for smelling by putting a pinch of cinnamon, nutmeg, clove, allspice, rosemary, thyme, or other favorites in a pill bottle. A cotton ball stuffed into the top keeps the spices in place when the top is opened.

They also suggest that visitors collect interesting photographs from magazines and advertisements. Mount them on cardboard and put them up. Change them often. They also recommend that you bring a masterpiece from a grandchild's kindergarten class, or birdseed to scatter outside a window, or fast-growing seeds to plant in a small, colorful pot (Griffith and Sandberg, 1982).

Chapter 7

Ministering to the Dying

OUR CONFLICTS WITH DEATH AND DYING

Sooner or later, if you continue to minister to the sick, you will work with someone who is dying. Don't panic. You have been around dying people all your life. Every day on earth moves each person closer to death, including you.

In the final analysis, there are only two major differences between the sick person who is dying and everybody else. The patient is sicker than most other people, and someone has made an educated guess about the amount of time before he or she will die.

Medical people usually want to save every life every time, and many dislike having to admit their limitations. They may feel they have failed their patient and his or her family when the patient dies. I've found it necessary on several occasions to remind medical doctors and nurses that, sooner or later, every patient they care for is going to die—it's just a matter of when. Nobody, however, wants the person to die on his or her watch.

When we face the dying person, most of us are facing far more. We are forced to remember our own mortality, the mortality of every person we love, and the deaths of others about whom we have cared. We may feel guilty because we will go on living after the person in front of us dies. Perhaps we secretly envy him or her for getting out of the troubles that life here on earth inevitably brings. Despite any and all the uncomfortable feelings we may experience when we face death with the person who is dying, we must respond to Jesus' command to love. We must deny ourselves the comfort that absence might afford and minister to the dying.

It is relatively easy for us to attend a Sunday school class, stand in the pulpit, or sit with a friend over a cup of coffee and talk about the fact that we are some day going to die. It is not easy, however, to sit at a bedside and talk with a person who is going to die within months, weeks, or days.

Having trained many ministers, I have concluded that most people want to believe there is some easy or correct thing to say when working with the dying. They believe that when they have learned that "secret something," working with the dying will not be so difficult. If you will quit looking for an easy way to conduct such a conversation, perhaps you will feel more at peace doing it. There is no easy way!

Perhaps we are looking at a perfect paradox—when we accept the fact that it isn't easy to discuss dying with a person who is dying, it becomes easier for us. I say this on the basis of having conducted hundreds of intimate conversations with people who were dying and having listened to experienced hospital chaplains for many years. Accept the fact that you are going to feel uncomfortable, and do it anyway. I believe this sort of action is a part of what Jesus was talking about when he told us to deny ourselves and to take up the cross and follow Him. When we work with the dying, we truly are denying ourselves the privilege of remaining comfortable. We give up or sacrifice our comfort for the sake of another. Love always costs the lover.

SOME FACTORS THAT INFLUENCE THE DYING PATIENT'S COPING PROCESS

Level of Awareness

The patient's process of coping and our ministry to the dying person will be influenced, in part, by everyone's level of awareness of the impending death. Because a hospital's laboratory tests are often conducted away from the hospital, a technician miles away is often the first to know that a patient is going to die. This early *limited awareness* remains even after the physician has read the report and also concluded that the patient is going to die. A *partial awareness* develops when the physician informs the nursing staff of the conclusion. A *suspected awareness* may then develop in the family or the patient.

Problems increase when the patient learns of the impending death but does not want the family to know. Alternatively, the family may learn of the impending death but does not want the patient to know. Sometimes the family knows and the patient knows, but the patient does not want the family to know that he or she knows, or the family does not want the patient to know that the family knows. Confusing? Yes. Complicated? Yes. Does it complicate our ministry to them? Yes! The patient and the family must decide how they want to handle it. We have no right to impose our opinion. Professional assistance by an adequately trained chaplain or other qualified person may help open dialogue that can benefit both the patient and the family.

Because a whole book would be required to discuss adequately all the possibilities implied in the foregoing paragraphs, I focus here only on ministering amid *open awareness* in which everyone involved knows that the patient is going to die (Glasser and Strauss, 1968).

Age and Level of Responsibility

The way people react to learning that they are going to die is influenced, in part, by their age and level of personal responsibility. A twenty-five-year-old mother with a child in elementary school and another in diapers will react differently from an eighty-five-year-old widow whose children are in their sixties. The younger person facing death usually will deal with feelings related to the loss of a future. The older person often will need to deal with feelings related to what could or should have been. Therefore, the more self-fulfilled the person is, the less difficulty he or she will experience in anticipation of death.

Individual Personality Traits

No two personalities are identical—not even the personalities of identical twins. No matter how similar people may be at times, each person's thoughts and experiences are unique. Our individual perspectives on life and death are unique. Therefore, while trying to cope with oncoming death, we may experience the five classic steps of denial, anger, bargaining, depression, and acceptance as described quite eloquently many years ago by Elisabeth Kübler-Ross (1969), but we may experience each step differently, and in no particular order, and some may never attain acceptance.

Cultural Differences

Each culture and subculture, somewhat unconsciously, establishes its own system of beliefs about life and death and the meaning of sickness and health. Some systems have a religious overtone. Others do not. One believes that all events are in the hands of a guided fate, and others believe all is in the hands of God. Still others believe that all is pure chance or that all events have a "purpose" or that all "just happens." One displays great emotion. Another stoically accepts without showing emotion. Everyone will have faced difficulties before, and we tend to fall back on that which has worked before.

Personal History

We all remember events. With the memories, we also retain the feelings associated with those events. We remember the people who have been important (positively and negatively) in our lives. We remember those we have harmed and those who have helped us. We recall our successes and failures, our tears and our laughter. We harbor memories and feelings related to the death of those we have loved.

A caring visitor will listen for comments that relate to the past and ask enough to encourage the patient to share those memories. Our ministry of listening requires that we give the patient opportunities for a life review of his or her successes and failures, joys and sorrows, good relationships and broken relationships. What has given meaning to your patient's life? The more at peace we become with the past, the more at peace we tend to be with the future. In what has your patient found the most satisfaction? The most frustration? What does he or she view as the most important lesson learned during the course of life? After you have listened to the things that have been voluntarily shared with you, you may even ask if your patient feels free to share life's greatest regrets. If your patient shares that with you, you must never repeat it to another soul as long as you live.

This kind of reminiscing sometimes brings back memories of strained or broken relationships that need reconciliation. Such issues can be catalogued under the heading of "unfinished business" that needs attention before one can die in peace.

All of this kind of conversation helps your patient to more comfortably close the door to this life. As this door is closed, you may sometimes get the feeling that the patient has begun to reach for the knob of the door that waits beyond.

After all that has been said, we must recognize that we human beings have no stereotypic response to our approach to death.

Anticipated Duration Before Death

People who know they are going to die within the next year will react differently from those who know they will be dying within a few weeks, days, or hours. The closer one gets to the death the less connected he or she may feel to those who have been close. Both the patient and those to whom he or she has been closely connected begin to disconnect. The dying person feels different. He or she feels less and less a sense of belonging. This difference and loss of belonging will accentuate the sense of distance in relationships.

The Personality Type

I have said that people tend to die as they have lived. Patients who are extroverted—outgoing, enjoying the company of others—tend to want others around them as they approach death. Those who have been somewhat introverted—preferring solitude and being concerned primarily with their own mental life—will be less interested in interacting with others in the face of death.

The Degree of Discomfort

People who are in excellent health tend to be the most frightened of death. Their fear is compounded by surprise—even shock. However unrealistic, young people tend to think that only older people become ill enough to die. On the other hand, many who are dying often look forward to death. Some may be road weary after a long, difficult trip through life. They may have endured so much pain and other discomforts that they want out—even if it means dying. Their spirit cries out, "Stop the world. I want to get off."

The Degree of Fulfillment of Life

The patient who has lived a fruitless, self-centered, meaning-less, unfulfilled life will face death much differently from the person who has lived a rich, spiritually and emotionally rewarding life. The former is likely to face death with regret, "I was given a great gift, life, but failed to use it well. I have wasted it." The latter is likely to face death with relative resolve and contentment. "I was given a great gift, life, and I have used it well."

Facing death, we tend to place on one side of a balance-scale all that the world and life has given us. On the other side we will place all that we have given back. Those who feel that the scales are tipped in favor of that which they have given will accept death more peacefully.

If you have experienced God's forgiveness, assure the patient of God's readiness to forgive.

The Religious Belief System

Beliefs about the nature of God, an after-death judgment of some sort, and possibilities of heaven or hell are among the many spiritual issues that color the response to impending death. I will discuss this later.

GOALS WHILE WORKING WITH THE DYING

A major goal for ministry to the sick is to provide *emotional and spiritual support* and to help patients to use their experience for *personal growth.*

Emotional and Spiritual Support

Many years ago, a patient flattered and frightened me when he said, "Chaplain, you seem to be a man with a lot of inner strength and a man of faith. I know I'm not going to be around much longer. I'm scared, and right now, my faith in God is pretty weak, too. I think I need to borrow your faith for a while."

We provide support by our physical presence. We probably provide the *best* support when we remain with the person from whom we feel most like running. If you see a quivering chin or moisture in the eyes *and* feel the person is trying to refrain from crying, he or she probably is trying not to cry.

Sometimes we provide support by telling a person that it's okay to cry. People are often more afraid of our condemnation than they are of God's. Therefore, we may need to give support by reassuring that it is all right to feel frightened or angry—at life or even at God.

People sometimes want to know that, despite all, nothing can separate them from the love of God (Rom. 8:39). You can assure them of this by saying it in prayers with your patient.

Although I have yet to understand all of the spiritual and emotional processes, I know that we give support by touching. Beware and be aware of your movements, but recognize that support is given and received by touching one another. A hand on the shoulder, a lingered firm handshake, and even a hug is often welcome.

(When my wife lay close to death from a cerebral hemorrhage, one evening I stood quietly sobbing just inside the door of the hospital's intensive care unit. I became aware of an arm firmly around my waist. I heard a whispered voice, "God loves you and cares about whatever is going on." This person cared that I was hurting, and, somewhere deep inside, I found reassurance that God cares. Perhaps it is true that suffering gains meaning only when the sufferer knows that someone cares [Lockerbie, 1998]. I had never seen this woman before that moment, and after she slipped out the door I never saw her again. She spoke reassuring words when I needed to hear them from outside myself. She dared to risk hugging me. She gave support! [All angels do not live in heaven— yet.])

Helping to Grow

Why would we want to help the person grow when we know he or she is dying? Is it a waste of time for us and a waste of energy for the patient?

My answer requires a statement of my personal belief system and you may or may not agree. I believe that after death, we who have lived in a trusting relationship with Christ as Lord and Savior will live in a place, state, or dimension that is beyond this world. I envision death as a door through which we pass to get from our current dimension of life into another. I also have difficulty imagining true life without some form of continuing growth.

Consider the example of a patient I will call Ms. Edwards. Ms. Edwards will be the same person on the other side that she was when she departed from this side. The more of her personality— her soul—her spirit that she will have developed on this side of death, the farther along she will be on the other side. Having taken advantage of opportunities for growth here, perhaps she will not have quite as far to grow before being able to fully receive and enjoy that which God holds in store for her.

We grow when we increase our faith. Your patient has experienced difficulties before this time. Did God help in any way during those times? If so, ask your patient to describe how. In doing so, his or her faith may be strengthened.

One person may grow by developing the courage not to commit suicide. Another may grow by developing the courage to surrender to death without a fight. Either attainment may be gained while engaging in quiet conversation with a fellow human being who is courageous enough to listen to the thoughts about such issues.

Many people drag around past injustices and failures as if they were links of a treasured golden chain when in reality they are worthless. A person has grown when he or she can say with the Apostle Paul, "forgetting those things which are behind, and reaching forth unto those things which are before, I press toward the mark for the prize of the high calling of God in Jesus Christ" (Phil. 3:13).

People grow when they forgive others and themselves and when they accept the forgiveness of others and of God. A decision to change attitudes and behaviors that help to improve relationships is growth for anyone at any time in life. People have truly grown when they recognize that they have the ability to cope with whatever the future holds: "If I live, I'm okay. If I die, I'm okay. I'm ready to deal with whatever life holds for me."

People move into peace with their coming death when they are given the privilege of reviewing their life story with one who is willing to listen without interruption or criticism. Someone has even given this a title: Life Review Therapy. To use this technique you don't need to be a therapist. You need only time and the determination to listen. Ask only enough questions to permit your patient to talk. Watch and listen to what happens when you say, "Ms. Edwards, I've got the time and you seem to have the energy. I'd enjoy hearing your story. Where did it all begin for you?" The moment she begins strolling along that wandering trail with you, she no longer feels alone. Somewhere deep inside, she gets the idea, "If this person is willing to walk with me through that long road of the past, perhaps God really is 'with' me as I take these final few steps. Because God cares more than my visitor does, maybe God really will walk with me *through* the valley of the shadow of death." When you look back on this sort of conversation, you may recognize that your work with the dying became work with life and living more than with death and dying.

If you are interrupted, the next time you visit, relax and remind her of what she was telling you when you were interrupted. "Ms. Edwards, when we were talking the last time, you were telling me about all those feelings you experienced when your first child was born"—or whatever she was telling you when she had to stop.

During her life review, she quite likely will tell you of some important truths she has learned along the way. In doing so, if she sees that she is teaching you from her experience, she is empowered by feeling that her life has meaning even while she is dying. You can add meaning to her life, even in the face of death, by asking a question. "Ms. Edwards, as you look back over your life, what do you think is the most important truth you have ever learned?" Thank her for sharing it with you. (Would we not receive a marvelous education if we learned the answer to that question of everyone we meet?)

Everything we have been thinking about relates to our willingness to actively listen and pray for the Holy Spirit of God to minister through us. I have trained too many laypeople to believe that the ministry we are discussing is only for the professional minister.

SHOULD THE PATIENT BE TOLD THAT HE OR SHE IS NEARING DEATH?

No matter what you may believe, and no matter how thoroughly you have thought through the issues, this is not a decision for you to make! I've listened to the debates of some of the most learned people, but no one has ever come up with an answer that works for everyone.

Ultimately, the decision to tell or not to tell the patient is a medical decision, made by the medical staff, based on what they believe to be best for their patient and the family at the time. However, it is quite appropriate for you to call the physician's office and ask permission to be present when he or she breaks the news to the patient and family (pastors and chaplains, please see the final section of this chapter).

WHAT CAN WE EXPECT OF THE PERSON WHO LEARNS THAT HE OR SHE IS SOON GOING TO DIE?

Shock and Depression

Followed by immediate denial, shock and depression are the most common first responses to learning of one's approaching death. I've concluded that the more abrupt the disclosure, the more profound the shock and depression. Of course, most people are in shock for a while, even if they already suspect that their illness is fatal. If the truth is simply more than Ms. Edwards can adjust to quickly, she probably will enter a period of denial.

Denial

Denial is used by almost all of us about almost anything we find emotionally unmanageable. We use this technique until we discover a way to cope with reality. Your patient may deny only long enough to think or say, "Oh no!" Or she may still be denying reality at the moment of death. Although most people seem to want to talk about their approaching death, the patient in denial may refuse to talk about it. If the patient speaks of the impending death at all, he or she may do so as if time were standing still. If the physician has specified a life expectancy of about a year, nine months later the patient still may be speaking of it as if it were twelve months away.

Whatever your beliefs about the importance of accepting reality, this is not the time to force the patient to face reality. As long as patients deny the issues, somewhere deep inside they know they do not yet have the inner resources for adequately coping.

Anger

Anger may soon follow the breakthrough of truth—I'm going to die! The anger may be directed at anything or anybody—including you. (If you catch a salvo of fury, refuse to take it personally.) Anger also may be generalized against life and the whole world. People may tell you that it does not make sense to them, but they feel angry toward every person they see and virtually everything they see. Although your patient has worked hard for forty years, he or she is losing everything.

Your patient is also being denied the privilege of completing goals. Even those who are 100 and of sound mind and body *still* have goals they hope to achieve and will be frustrated not to accomplish them. Such frustrated people will find a target for their anger.

The medical staff makes a good target. After all, Ms. Edwards or her insurance company is paying them good money to make her well. Not only are her doctors and the hospital staff failing to repair her, they are letting her die.

Ms. Edwards may turn her anger against herself. All her life, her body has done as her mind has told it to do. She has said, "Foot, move," and it has moved. "Hand, move," and it has moved as she has directed. Now she may feel that her body has turned against its master, refusing to follow orders. If she knows she has contributed to her own decline of health, the anger against herself may be more intensified. Perhaps she has smoked cigarettes for years, or she has consistently eaten unhealthy foods, or she has watched a growing lump and failed to call it to the attention of her physician.

If she cannot find anyone else with whom to feel angry, she may turn her anger against God. The belief that God gives health and wealth to good people and sickness and poverty to evil people is as alive today across the United States as it was in the Middle East in the days of Job.

God is commonly viewed as a heavenly bully who pushes people around, giving them such disasters as cancer and heart disease, and causing accidents for themselves, their children, or other loved ones. He is commonly viewed as the "grand killer" who ultimately takes every life. If you believe someone, anyone, even God, is about to kill you, you are likely to feel anger toward him.

If you feel anger toward God, and admit it to yourself, you might feel quite frightened. All of your life, you have watched a common human practice. When Carol has become angry with Beverly, Beverly has automatically become angry with Carol. Therefore, if your patient feels anger toward God, he or she may think, "Oh no! I'm about to die. And I'm going to have to face God for judgment. My judge is going to know I've been angry with him. *I've had it!* I may be in danger of being sent directly into the most terrible corner of hell!"

If Ms. Edwards is one who dreads God's condemnation, you do not need to add your condemnation to her troubled mind. She needs your love and acceptance. Remind her that *nothing* can separate her from the love of God (Rom. 8:39). We don't have to defend God. If God is so threatened by the anger of a mere mortal, the human race is in deep trouble. Unless someone reminds Ms. Edwards, she may not remember that her anger places her in the company of some tall figures in the Bible. Who can fail to hear the anger of the writer of the forty-fourth psalm when he believes God is uncaring and sleeping through the troubles of his people? Can we not hear the anger of the prophet Jeremiah when God had permitted his enemies to imprison him in a pit (Jer. 20:7-18)? Instead of criticizing your patient's tottering faith and anger, remind him or her that our Lord Jesus, the earthly personification of God, demonstrated that love absorbs anger and does not retaliate in kind.

Fear of Death

The fear of death is far more prevalent in those who are well than in those who are ill. Those who are "up and around," going about their normal activities of work, play, and sleep, are most afraid of death. As I have listened, I have concluded that most people are not so much afraid of death as they are afraid of dying. Dying is the process we go through before we die. Most people are frightened by thoughts of pain, suffering, indignities, helplessness, and all that we can go through before arriving at death.

The extremely ill person is already experiencing much that the dying person may experience and many hold no fear of death. They want out. Many are eager to get out.

Although Ms. Edwards may sincerely trust Christ as her Lord, she may still fear death. Christianity is based on faith. In part, the Christian faith is a belief system without personal experiential knowledge. "Yes," she may say, "Jesus arose from the dead. But will I?" Most of us can identify, at least to some degree, with the struggling man who once said to Jesus, "I believe, but help thou my unbelief" (Mark 9:24). Most people believe the adage, "a bird in the hand is worth two in the bush." They know what they have now, but they do not absolutely know what is on the other side.

Christians are not alone in believing in an afterlife. People of many faiths and cultures have believed for centuries in some form of life after death. To this day, we recognize that whatever the religion, those of deep faith tend to die with less fear than those of no faith or shallow faith. The atheist will tell you that such a benefit of faith for the dying is only a psychological mechanism that comforts the mind. Of course, comfort has a psychological dimension, but not all comes from within. The answers to questions may be found in eternity.

Faith can be shared. Let others borrow from your faith if they are courageous enough to tell you of their moments of doubt. Telling them they "should not feel that way" will not change their feelings or their thoughts. Such words will only add to their pain. Re-assure them that despite their questions and even their doubts, our Lord still loves them.

The Feeling of Separation

Feeling separated is the natural companion to feeling different. If Ms. Edwards is dying, not only does she *feel* different, she *is* different. She *knows* that she will die soon. Encourage her family to include her in as much of their activity as possible. Include her in as much conversation as possible. If she cannot talk, do not talk as if she were not there. You might play cards, checkers, or some other game with her. If she is putting together a jigsaw puzzle, find a few pieces and put them in place. I've experienced a sense of closeness with patients over checkerboards and jigsaw puzzles when all previous visits have seemed distant.

If you have any suspicion that she is feeling separated from those with whom she has formerly felt close, you may once again refer her to Romans 8:38-39. Not even death can separate her from the love of God in Christ.

Depression

Depression comes and goes throughout the period of decline as the patient progresses toward death. Almost everything discussed in this chapter may contribute to his or her depression. We must remember that suicide is always a possible response of your patient as long as he or she has the capability.

This possibility may terrify you, but we learned long ago that caring, informed laypeople often are more effective in dissuading from suicide than professionals. Your genuine heartfelt love, your concern, your compassion, your listening ear, your refusal to criticize, your honest humanity that admits that you, too, might want to die if you were facing the same issues—these are your most effective tools when working with the suicidal person.

Yes, your words that reassure the ongoing presence and compassion of Jesus are valuable. Beware, however, of the temptation to give rehearsed answers to your patient's struggles. "Pat" answers to profound questions help no one. Indeed, they tend to add to the sense of frustration and anger.

If you get the impression that Ms. Edwards may be considering suicide, ask her. Don't worry about planting the idea or causing her to do it by your inquiry. She may speak of "not waiting" or "getting it over with." She may speak of refusing to let the doctors or hospitals get all she has planned to leave her family. If she speaks as if she is considering revenge against someone close to her, suspect thoughts of suicide. If she speaks of intense anger against herself, that may be a clue to her thoughts.

Listen to the language. Does she speak passively or actively? People who speak of wanting to die are far less likely to kill themselves than those who admit that they are thinking about ending it all. One is passive. The other is active. One *wants* something to happen. The other is thinking of *making* something happen.

If she talks of doing something to kill herself, ask how she would do it. Does she have the *ability* and the *means* to do what she tells you? If she wants to jump off a tall building, but can't get out of bed, obviously the ability and means reduce the probability. However, if she wants to shoot herself and has a .38 revolver in the bedside table, the probability is high.

Remind the patient of the legacy he or she will leave behind. Family and friends will feel guilty. For many years, they will ask themselves how they might have kept their loved one from commiting suicide. Those who kill themselves leave behind a model of behavior: When things get tough, kill yourself. Descendants of those who have killed themselves, statistically, are more likely to kill themselves than others.

If your patient admits to having decided on a suicide method, ask him or her to promise (preferably in writing) to call you or some other support person before taking action. You might also ask the person to make an appointment with you at some time beyond which you think the action might be taken.

Under such conditions, when suicidal people have refused to make an appointment with me, I have made the appointment with them. "Even though you won't promise not to kill yourself tonight, I am going to call you tomorrow morning at ten o'clock." (You set the time.) Be sure to call! The feeling that at least one person cares if he or she lives or dies can make the difference between life and death.

Then *tell the patient's physician.* Having worked with families of many dozens of people who have killed themselves, I learned long ago that family members do not want to believe that their loved ones would actually kill themselves. When I was working to help establish a suicide prevention service, I learned that about 75 percent of those who kill themselves have told someone within twenty-four hours of the act.

If your patient commits suicide, it is not your fault! It is that person's decision. You are headed into deep trouble the moment you begin accepting responsibility for other people's choices. Having been educated in the field of "suicidology" and having worked with hundreds of people who were suicidal, long ago I arrived at a conclusion. No matter how well trained, or skillful, or knowledgeable, or fluent in language we may be, we cannot stop someone who has fully decided to commit suicide.

Our greatest impact is made while the decision is pending. We can demonstrate our care, our concern, our compassion, our love, and sometimes our tears as we listen with hope that he or she will refrain from self-slaughter. This is another time that we will hope and pray that our Lord and his love will be radiated through us.

Bargaining with God or Fate or Life

Bargaining is common for the person facing death. "If I get well, I will . . ." The promise may be made to God, to a mate, or to a friend, or it may be made to you. Take it seriously. If the patient recovers, he or she may or may not follow through with the commitment. Bargaining often arises from feelings of guilt. "Because I have done as I should not have done, or I have failed to do as I should have done, if I recover I will do as I should have been already doing."

Guilt

Guilt will contribute to your patient's depression. One day Ms. Edwards may look at you, or her husband (whom she loves), or her child (also whom she loves) and for a fleeting moment she may think, "I wish you were dying instead of me." Then she condemns herself!

Of course, as she declines, she is likely to have reflected on her past. She may look at her successes, but she will also review her failures and her regrets. Although some of these regrets may result from major blunders she's made in her life, even the small things often take on significance. I recall a man who confessed to a failure that might be considered insignificant. He had been visiting an old man in a nursing home whose eyeglasses were terribly smudged. He neglected to follow the impulse to offer to clean them. Twenty years later, he was feeling guilty for his neglect. This may be a small matter, but when Jesus said, "I was thirsty and you gave me no drink" (Matthew 25:42), that seemed like a small matter, too. (Perhaps my patient was reminding me that in God's eyes, the small things that make up our everyday lives truly are big things.)

Keep in mind that when Ms. Edwards makes such an admission of a failure, she is confessing! She is following scriptural instruction: "*Confess* your faults to one another, and *pray for one another* that you may be healed" (James 5:16). The healing may be to the soul, not necessarily to the body. Such a confession may be made in your presence, but it is more truly made to God who is in the room with you. You stand on holy ground. Reverence the experience with secrecy. Talk with no one but our Lord about what you have heard.

It would not be unusual for Ms. Edwards to also feel guilty for the emotional and financial drain she thinks her condition may be imposing on her family. She may not know the exact figures, but she probably knows that her illness is costing more than $600 per day just for the room charge. Even the best insurance probably will not pay all. She may also feel terribly guilty for leaving her family to pay the medical bills, as well as the emotional high cost of loving her.

Guilt has only one emotional and spiritual solution. The solution is forgiveness. Here is your opportunity to speak as a prophet—spokesperson for our Lord. You do not need to declare, "Thus saith the Lord," but if you are confident that God loves her and wants to forgive her, tell her. Tell your patient that God loves her despite all of her guilt, and, if she will accept forgiveness, God forgives her.

Acceptance

The person who can live at peace with approaching death has found acceptance. During this period, we may erroneously conclude that all is well. It is. At least, all is well for that particular moment. A few minutes later, however, he or she may be back at any of the stages already discussed. Therefore, we must deal with patients where we find them instead of trying to relate to them as they were at a prior time or where we think they may be tomorrow.

During the process of adjustment you may encourage Ms. Edwards to say some things that will help her to find peace. Because they are obvious, I will simply list five without comment. She will find additional peace by saying to the appropriate person or persons

1. Forgive me.
2. I forgive you.

3. Thank you.
4. I love you.
5. Good-bye.

While in a state of acceptance, patients may decrease activities in order to preserve energy for living. Conversely, they may become so overly active that they hasten their death.

Someone who accepts death might ask you to do something that may tax your greatest courage. If Ms. Edwards is in extreme, unrelieved pain, has ongoing nausea or some other major discomfort, she might ask you to pray for God to hasten her death. Some patients simply grow weary of struggling. The last words my grandmother spoke to me were, "I'm tired. I want to go home." I decided long ago that if a person has the courage to ask me to pray for God to relieve them by death, I will find the courage to do as he or she asks.

Only you can make your own decision about what to do. Having honored such requests, I cannot say that I ever did so without deep personal distress. If you have a quiver in your voice while you pray such a prayer, that's okay. Your patient probably knows that his or her request places a burden upon you and will make it somewhat apologetically. If you comply, be prepared for the warmest "Thank you" that you have ever received.

Loneliness

Loneliness tends to be a major cause of depression for the dying. In a modern hospital with a thousand or more employees and several hundred patients with visiting families coming and going, why would the dying person feel lonely? Many have confirmed that they feel loneliest in a crowd.

Some will emotionally detach from their family as a way of trying to protect those they love. However, during the process of dying, each person needs the warmth and closeness of other human beings. Unfortunately, the dying person often is forced to die alone—abandoned.

Many tend to distance themselves from the dying person. Studies have shown that friends visit less often after they learn of impending death. When they do visit, they spend less time. Other studies have concluded that even doctors and nurses spend less time with their patients after they learn the patient is dying. Maybe they don't know what to say. People fear saying the wrong thing. Our patient may remind us of our own mortality or the mortality of our loved ones. Perhaps we dislike feeling helpless in the patient's presence. The point is, the dying person tends to be left to die alone.

Almost every patient who enters a hospital thinks about the possibility of dying. The distancing typically begins the first time the patient brings up the subject. If patients initiate the subject of possible death, give them a chance to talk about it! Your patient may be in the hospital for a broken foot, but almost anything can be going on in his or her mind. For instance, your patient might say, "I don't think I am going to get well this time" or "I think I may never get out of the hospital." If patients say anything that makes you think that they believe they may die, let them talk! Even encourage them to talk.

If you can think fast enough to make a statement instead of asking a question, you might say, "Tom, you sound as if you think you may die." If you are incorrect, you have said nothing wrong. If you are right, sit back and listen.

If you can only ask a question, you might ask, "Tom, are you saying that you believe you are going to die?" or "What feelings do you have when you think about dying?"

About the only wrong thing you can say is that which almost everybody else is likely to say to him: "Oh, don't talk like that. You will probably outlive all of us." He is likely to hear this from his family and his closest friends. Don't let him hear it from his minister. When we respond in that fashion, we have effectively said,

"Hush! I don't have the courage to face this with you. I don't want to hear what you have to say about it." If he hears this sort of response a couple of times, he is likely to conclude, "Nobody wants to hear me. I guess I'll have to walk through the valley of the shadow of death alone." I wish I did not believe what I am telling you, but I have heard it so often that I cannot believe otherwise.

This means that in an institution populated with hundreds of people there are people in danger of dying alone. The dying have reason to feel that people are avoiding spending time with them, and those who do spend time with them are putting more and more emotional distance between them. Christians can, again, learn from the Jews. They believe no person should die alone.

If you have determined to see it through to the end with your patient, stand or sit close to his bed. Let your patient talk about anything he or she chooses, and then listen. Sometimes sit with your patient in silence. The patient is aware of your presence. Silence is awkward only to those who feel like talking. Look for an opportunity for a gentle touch to the hand or arm. You don't want the patient's only touch to be from a nurse injecting medicine. You might even ask if your patient would feel comfortable receiving a hug.

Heightened Sense of Hearing

While the rest of the body is shutting down, the sense of hearing in some dying people sometimes improves. Therefore, even if the patient is not in a coma, follow the guidelines for ministering to the comatose patient offered in Chapter 8.

Grief

Grief is that complex set of emotions experienced at the loss of a person or thing that is loved. Notice that I did not define grief as an emotion but as a complex set of emotions. This set includes sadness, anger, guilt, confusion, and anxiety. Some think of the coming and going of these emotions as cyclical or as grief attacks. One attack may feel somewhat easy to manage, but another may follow that is almost overwhelming. I usually think of them as the waves upon a beach. The feelings don't always make sense. They are "just there," and when they have gone, they are likely to return. We may not know from where they came, and we can say with less certainty where they have gone. All of these waves of grief are accompanied by memories of the past and thoughts of what will be lost in the future. These thoughts and feelings make up the process of adjustment and movement toward peace with that which has been, or is being lost.

We understand that the patient's family will begin to grieve as soon as they learn of the impending death. We even have a name for it. We call it anticipatory grief—grief that begins before a death in anticipation of the coming loss of the person in whom we have held an emotional investment.

As you work with the dying, remember that the patient's grief may be far more profound and more complicated than the grief of the family. If I were to learn tomorrow that I will die in the near future, my wife would begin preparing to lose one husband. My son and daughter would each be preparing to lose one father. My son-in-law would be preparing to lose one father-in-law. Each of my few friends would be preparing to lose one friend. As long as they remain on Earth, we will never interrelate again.

I, however, would be losing my wife, my son and daughter, my son-in-law, and each person I consider a friend. Therefore, the dying person's grief may be much more profound than that of the family and other loved ones.

This may be just as true of the Christian as of the non-Christian. You may have heard someone suggest, "Because we trust Christ as Lord and Savior, we should not mind dying. We are going to heaven and we will get to be with him! Therefore the true Christian should not dread dying as much as the non-Christian." However, I have reason to believe that the Christian who is losing a family member to death may sometimes hurt more than the nonbeliever. I also believe I know why.

Having watched and having been a professional listener for many years, I have concluded that people whose lives are committed to Christ tend to love more deeply than the others do. I wish someone would do some research on this matter. Perhaps I speak only a biased, though educated, opinion.

The more deeply we love someone, the more deeply we feel the pain when that person is gone. Despite the faith and hope we hold in expectation of a reunion with loved ones in a heavenly afterlife, the dying person knows that he or she is losing them for as long as they remain alive. Dying people also hurt because they know that the people who love them are hurting.

DEATHBED REPENTANCES

Before I continue, I want to assure you that I have a vital concern for both the temporal welfare and the eternal welfare of those to whom you and I minister. On many occasions, I have rejoiced at the privilege of having given witness to the redemptive, re-creative power of God in human life—but *rarely* have I seen it with the dying.

With few extremely rare exceptions, *people die as they have lived.* Those who have lived their lives trusting Christ as Lord and Savior tend to die trusting Christ as Lord and Savior. On some occasions, I have listened quietly to my patients who seemed to be "coming and going" while speaking with excitement of the beauty they could see "on the other side."

Those who have lived their lives without trusting Christ as Lord and Savior tend to die without trusting Christ as Lord and Savior. At the end some have cried that they were burning and tormented by demons. I remember one who died screaming, "Oh, God! The flames! The flames!"

In my young years, I heard many ministers tell stories of "death-bed repentances." I heard so many of them that I assumed it was common for gospel ministers to hear first-time professions of Christian faith by people in their final days, hours, or minutes. I no longer believe this. During my thirty-one years of hospital ministry, I was privileged to develop friendships and warm acquaintances with several hundred evangelical ministers. I have chatted with ministers on many occasions shortly after they had visited with the hospitalized sick of their communities. I have heard them tell of no more than ten or twelve deathbed repentances. When I quizzed other hospital chaplains on the subject, they have had similar experiences.

From where, then, do all of those stories come? I think I know. Reverend Jones visits a man who is dying. In the course of his ministry, the patient confesses Christ as Lord. Reverend Jones rejoices as he tells the story at the weekly, monthly, or annual meeting of the pastor's conference. From a dozen to several hundred ministers hear the story. Many of those then weave the story into a sermon within the next few weeks. Each listening congregation concludes that the minister is speaking of his own experience. A hundred ministers ultimately may tell the story of the one death-bed repentance, and each of their congregations will have concluded that the conversion has been the result of the ministry of the minister who is speaking.

Does all that I've been saying mean that we will make no effort to evangelize the dying person? No! However, we will *beware of manipulating dying people into saying words we want to hear them say.* If I can stir enough fear within the dying person, I suspect I could get him or her to say almost anything that I want to hear. However, the ethics and morality of doing so must be seriously questioned!

TRUST IN YOURSELF AND YOUR RESOURCES

I hope you have not become frightened or discouraged by all that you have read in this book. Courage is not the lack of fear. Courage is in the movement forward while fear churns within your breast. Go lovingly into the world of the sick and enjoy God's blessing and people's gratitude.

As you go, use your resources. Your patient is under the care of professional people. My work has given me the privilege of working with many nurses, and I feel proud to identify myself with a respected body of men and women known as hospital chaplains. To prepare themselves for this ministry, most of them have undergone one to three years of specialized training (a chaplaincy internship and possibly a residency program) beyond their bachelor's degree and beyond a three-year master's degree from a theological seminary.

You probably have one of these people on the staff of your local hospital. Use that person as your professional consultant. No one in your community is more qualified to respond to your questions or concerns about ministering to the sick and/or the dying. Please be patient and forgive the chaplain if he or she is called away to the scene of an emergency.

ADVICE FOR PASTORS
AND PROFESSIONAL HOSPITAL CHAPLAINS

The remaining pages of this chapter are intended for pastors and those persons who are in training to become professional hospital chaplains.

In the course of my ministry as a hospital chaplain, I have known many doctors. I have never known one, however, who seemed truly comfortable in giving news of impending death to the patient or family. Many are looking for all the help they can get.

If you suspect that the patient is going to die, you have an opportunity to enhance your interprofessional relationships by calling the patient's primary physician. Identify yourself to the doctor's receptionist and ask to speak to the doctor in reference to "Ms. Edwards" (name the specific patient). Tell the doctor that you suspect that your patient may soon die. Tell the doctor *that if he or she wants,* you will be willing to be present when the bad news is given.

Some doctors have wanted me there, and we have met at an appointed time and place. Before going into the room, clarify expectations. Does the physician want to be present to answer medical questions after you have given the bad news, or does he or she want to give the information and then leave you to minister? You do not want to walk in and stand there with each of you expecting the other to give the bad news. Other doctors have wanted me there but preferred that I enter shortly after they have given the news. Of course, this, too, requires an appointment to be set with the physician.

When we have met at the appointed time and place, I have asked, "Tell me exactly how long I should wait after you have gone in before I knock on the door." The usual suggestion has been for me to wait three minutes (sometimes four or five). Time it. If the physician indicates three minutes, knock on the door *exactly* three minutes after he or she has gone into the room. After you enter, you can expect the doctor to leave soon, letting you remain with the upset patient and family (and probably glad to get out of the room). This is one of those times when you probably will not leave within that ten-minute period I suggested earlier. You will stay and *listen* to the patient and family *as long as they seem to feel the need* to talk about pertinent issues. You must do ten times more listening than talking at this time.

Some doctors will prefer you to enter the room with them. Listen carefully to every word the doctor tells the patient and family. Because people are in such a state of shock upon hearing the bad news, they may hear nothing the doctor then says about options, or treatment, or the course that the illness is likely to take. You will be listening while the doctor is talking so that, if needed later, you can repeat what the doctor has said. You may also write the unanswered questions for them to read to the physician when he or she returns.

Also, while the doctor is talking, if you do not understand the medical language he or she is using, assume that the family also does not understand. Doctors and nurses often get so caught up in medical details that they forget they are using professional medical jargon. Never has a doctor become impatient when I have politely interrupted, saying "Sorry, Doctor. I'm not sure I understood the meaning of that word or phrase you used. If I didn't understand, they too might not have understood."

This kind of ministry requires that you return and visit again with this patient approximately twenty-four hours later. Not only will you have built a significant bond with the patient and family, but the next time you see that physician he or she probably will greet you as a long lost friend. You will be recognized as a member of *their* team.

Chapter 8

Ministering to Other Difficult Patients

Even if you have years of experience in ministering to the sick, you may sometimes see a name on your sick list that stirs a sense of dread. You well remember prior visits with that person. You may not have known what to do or what to say. You secretly know that the sense of dread is created by feelings of inadequacy. You probably have never told anyone of such feelings because you also felt both guilty and ashamed of them.

You may even feel that a ministry to some of the people you are supposed to serve is a waste of time. You feel so loaded with responsibility that you have no time to waste. If you feel like running from the "impossible" person, it may be because he or she reminds you of the condition you, or someone you love, may someday experience or have experienced in the past. Ask our Lord to help you to find the courage to endure the discomfort long enough to minister to such people. Ministry may appear impossible when it is only difficult.

MINISTERING TO THE COMATOSE PATIENT

You might feel that it is senseless to minister to the comatose patient. The coma may be the result of any of a number of physical problems: a serious head injury received in an accident or a massive stroke. Stroke patients present the greatest problem for many who would minister to them.

There are two kinds of stroke. The most common type occurs when a blood vessel in the brain has become closed off by a thrombus (a blood clot). The clot may have formed in the brain, or it may have been part of a larger clot that formed elsewhere in the body that broke off, moved, and became lodged in a narrowed segment of a blood vessel of the brain. This kind of stroke often causes death a few days after the event or leaves the patient severely paralyzed and unable to speak. Such patients may cry whenever a visitor enters their room. You haven't done anything wrong. They are frightened, frustrated, or angry. All three emotions can result in tears. Reassure them that it is all right with you if they cry and that doing so may possibly help them. Then sit quietly while they continue.

The other type of stroke, the cerebral hemorrhage, is a bleed within the brain tissue itself. This bleed results from some trauma that has torn open a blood vessel or from a ruptured aneurysm (a ruptured weak place in a blood vessel). Some people acquire this weakness over time, and others live with this time bomb congenital weakness from birth. A cerebral hemorrhage also may occur when a blood vessel ruptures and releases blood into the brain because of accelerated hypertension. The cerebral hemorrhage often kills instantly. However, if the patient survives the initial assault to the brain, every minute of survival slightly increases the statistical probability of a full recovery.

The risk of death from stroke is greatest within the first forty-eight to seventy-two hours. If your patient survives those first few days he or she probably will show slow but steady improvement. Some recover completely with no residual difficulties. However, a high percentage experience long-term neurological deficiencies.

You sometimes will hear both types of stroke called a *cerebral vascular accident* (CVA). However, because the public is so familiar with heart attacks, *brain attack* is becoming the preferred term.

(Coincidentally, while I wrote these lines, I was 500 miles from home. My wife and I were in Panama City, Florida, on vacation, when she experienced a cerebral hemorrhage and was placed in an intensive care unit. My wife seems to have recovered completely.)

Whether from a stroke, an accidental blow on the head, a brain tumor, or any other cause, your patient may become comatose. Patients in a coma may appear to be totally unconscious—totally unaware of anything or anybody. Someone (even a member of the medical staff) may have said of the patient, "He doesn't know he is in the world."

Having served as a full-time, professional hospital chaplain at the bedside for thirty-one years, I tell you not to believe those words—no matter who speaks them. *The person in a coma sometimes can hear every word said in his or her presence.* I would need far more words than I've allotted for this whole chapter to tell you my many war stories about what people have told me they heard while in the depths of a coma.

I'll briefly tell you one that illustrates the issue for thousands. While teaching a college-level course titled Ministering to the Sick, I said to the class, "Although you may have been told that your patient is in a coma, unaware of anything, always assume that the coma patient can hear every word you speak." A student's hand shot up.

"Chaplain, I can tell you all about that. A few years ago, I was in a car wreck and in a coma for more than a week. During that time, I heard the doctors talking about tickling my feet and sticking me with pins, trying to see if I would respond. They talked about my head injury and about the many broken bones I had. Physically, I felt nothing. But I could think, and emotionally I could feel everything. It was as if I was suspended in space—a mind without a body. I was *terrified* when I heard them say that I didn't have a chance to live. And I was angry that they were thoughtless enough to say those kinds of things around me."

If you *always assume that your comatose patients can hear every word you say,* you may quickly recognize the possibility of performing a much-needed ministry. When you walk into their presence, speak to them. If you know of people who are praying for them and their family, tell them. Bring them news of things going on at church (positive news only) and of community or sports events. When a person is in that never-never land, feeling isolated and lost in space, the knowledge that someone cares enough to bring news from home is uplifting and stimulating. This promotes healing and encourages the fight to recover.

In the comatose condition, their minds may be too confused—too foggy to put into words even a silent prayer. Therefore, when you pray, pray aloud. If they can hear, they can make your prayer their own. Let them hear you praying for their family, too.

MINISTERING TO THE ALZHEIMER'S PATIENT

Just the mention of Alzheimer's disease may flood you with a wave of sadness. Perhaps you feel a black terror—or is it both? You probably are uncomfortable visiting with the family of the Alzheimer's victim and even more uncomfortable visiting with the patient. The illness may run in your own family, or someone else close to you may have it.

Alzheimer's is a progressive, degenerative disease of the brain characterized by confusion, loss of memory, disorientation, restlessness, speech disturbances, inability to carry out purposeful movements, and hallucinations. It usually strikes people after age sixty-five, but occasionally it affects some as young as thirty.

Authorities estimate that Alzheimer's disease now claims more than 2.5 million victims in the United States. Because of what I observed during my ministry on a geropsychiatric unit, I made a promise to myself: If any of my family were ever diagnosed with Alzheimer's disease, I would immediately ask for a referral for another opinion. I would get an evaluation by a gerontologist or a geropsychiatrist (both are a type of medical doctor who specializes in problems of people age sixty-five and older). Improper diet, medicines, and other correctable problems account for as much as 70 percent of the errors in diagnosis of Alzheimer's disease.

Alzheimer's annual financial burden in terms of cost of care and lost productivity is estimated to surpass 100 billion dollars a year (www.alzheimers.com). This relates only to the patients. Who would dare to estimate the emotional cost to the millions of family members and friends whose lives are also changed by their loved one's disease? The church must minister to all: the patient, the patient's family, and the patient's friends. The odds are high that some of the disease's victims are among those to whom you are called to minister.

You may remember when such patients were highly active, able to enjoy a good laugh, and could converse intelligently on almost any subject. The past few times you have visited them, however, they have cried. That's okay. Let them cry. They're probably frustrated by their disabilities and terrified by the future. Their tears are normal and healthy. Perhaps they show absolutely no emotion. They may just sit in one position for hours, staring into space.

Although their bodies may sit or lie in front of you, they seem to have gone somewhere else. They may not look at you even if you sit directly in front of them. Instead, they seem to look right through you. You speak but you get no response. You suspect they are not in touch with anything in this world. Is it possible to minister to them? Maybe. Maybe not.

Sometimes, you may find that God has ministered through you when you did not even know it. In the presence of impossible situations, you may sometimes feel that your cup does not "runneth over." Indeed, it may seem *empty,* and we may feel totally inadequate.

When we realize that we are completely inadequate, we generally do one of two things. We do nothing, or we depend on the One who is all adequate. We can ask our Lord to minister through us. The sooner we recognize that there are instances in which *no hu-*

man is adequate, the sooner we can more confidently accept our ministry to people in impossible situations. When a small child bleeds to death in his mother's arms, who is adequate to minister to all her needs? When an old man sees his wife instantly killed by a careless automobile driver, who is adequate to minister to all his needs? When a young man drowns while on his honeymoon, who is adequate to minister to all the grieving bride's needs? *Only* God.

The Apostle Paul made a statement on which all who minister would do well to ponder. "I live; yet not I, but Christ liveth in me" (Gal. 2:20). Even if the scriptures did not teach that Christ lives within us, I would suspect it on the basis of repeated personal experiences in my ministry as a hospital chaplain. One example will suffice.

I had been called to the scene after a man had been given terrible news concerning his wife's cancer. I introduced myself and sat down as he began to talk. In his anxiety, he spoke nonstop for at least forty-five minutes while I occasionally nodded my head and silently listened. I offered a brief prayer and left. The next day, walking with another minister, I met the man and asked about his wife. After he told of her latest condition, he turned to my minister friend and said, "Chaplain Justice will never know how encouraging his words were to me as we talked yesterday." I stood astonished. I had said almost nothing. Who had spoken those comforting words to him? Someone did! Because I had said almost nothing, I can only conclude that our Lord who lives within me (and him) had spoken to him so clearly while I was there that he assumed it had been I. I've had too many of these experiences to take them lightly.

When you are with the Alzheimer's patient or any number of others with whom you feel inadequate and that ministry by you is impossible, rely on the One who can minister through you—even to one who may seem to have mentally gone away. When you visit someone who has Alzheimer's, you may think you are seeing the person you might have known for many years. Instead, you are seeing only the face of the person you have known. The person you have known is gone. The person the family has loved is gone. (They may need you to remind them of that.) He or she has been replaced by a poor reflection of the one who once was.

The patient may have been progressively reduced to the level of a two-year-old child, but he or she is bigger and stronger and heavier and probably far more difficult to control than a child. These patients are often confused, frightened, and angered by people's actions and words—rarely understanding that anything has happened to them. To themselves, they are okay. It's the rest of the world that is acting strangely. Do not permit yourself to take it personally if the Alzheimer's victim lashes out at you with senseless accusations and insults. Never, never argue with Alzheimer's patients. They will only become agitated, and you will never see positive results!

They may follow the caregiver around like a puppy one day and wander across town the next. As their disease progresses, their world diminishes. You may remind the family of this. A walk around the block may be good exercise for the patients and for you. As you walk, focus on what is going on around you at the moment. This may also give a few moments of much-needed relief to the family.

No words in any language can describe the pain, the drain, and the strain experienced by the family of the Alzheimer's patient. Look into the eyes of the caregiving family and you will see indescribable sadness and exhaustion. Most get little or no relief. If you listen, some will tell you that they now find it easier to believe in a semi-living eternal hell. Even here on earth, their own suffering goes on and on with no end in sight. Many begin to experience moments in which they secretly wish their loved one would die. A moment later they feel hideously guilty. They need a ministry. They need relief.

Every church with a member who has Alzheimer's disease should examine the need for an organized respite ministry. In such a program, teams made up of a husband and wife, or two men, or two women visit in the patient's home each week, giving the family caregiver time to get away for a few hours. (For obvious reasons, men sit with male patients and women sit with female patients.) The family should be encouraged to do anything they want during this time. One may go shopping. Another may go and sit in a park. Another may go to a football game. The family should be encouraged to do something that will distract them from their cares at home.

When you visit with Alzheimer's patients, talk to them as if they hear and understand every word. They might and you may never know it. Although the short-term memory may be seriously damaged, the long-term memory may be quite intact. I have watched people who have seemed totally noncommunicative change suddenly when given an opportunity to join in the singing of an old song. "What's your favorite old hymn?" If named, I've asked many times, "Would you enjoy singing it with me?" Then enjoy it! Those who have been skilled in the playing of musical instruments often retain their skills much longer than their caregivers expect. A visitor's encouragement to exercise those residual talents may produce a surprising spring of joy for the patient and the family— and possibly for you too.

Some authorities who work consistently with elders praise the value of reminiscent therapy for the vast majority of senior citizens. Talking about past events, failures, and accomplishments seems to help them live more in peace with the past. The more at peace we are with our past, the more peace we may enjoy in the future. We experiment when we are trying to minister under such difficult circumstances. Patients who do not respond to your inquiry may have lost their pasts too. It may have been erased from the brain or blocked from access by the disease. Therefore, we may need to avoid talking about the past, and the family may need to be reminded that talking about past experiences may add to the patient's confusion.

However, people who have forgotten most events of years gone by may yet hold vivid memories from childhood. Ask your patients to tell you about those memories. "What is the first thing you recall from your childhood?" "What sort of things did you do with your mother [or sibling] when you were little?" "What kind of toys did you play with?" If your patient attended church activities in childhood, "Could you tell me about your first Sunday school teacher?" "What was the old church-house like when you were a child?" Then sit back and listen. Active listening can serve as a beneficial form of ministry.

If your patient is reduced to the level of the two-year-old, focus on the present—the piece of cake on the table, or the music in the background, or the animal program on TV.

I have long been fascinated by the power of the loving human touch. I am convinced that some form of energy often is transferred from one person to another by touching. Jesus appears to have been so sensitive that he once felt energy transfer from him to a woman who had touched merely the hem of his garment (Mark 5:25-34). Down through the years, people have recognized some kind of power in human touch. If you have been ordained for some office of your church, try to describe what you felt while hands were being placed on your head. You are likely to run out of words. The New Testament mentions the "laying on of hands" on several occasions. (Was that practice intended only as a ritual, or was it encouraged in normal interactions between human beings?) Pats on the back, a hug, and holding hands are often calming gestures, and they often communicate love and safety in a way even incapacitated people can understand.

If all of these problems related to Alzheimer's disease are uncomfortable for you, consider the caregivers who are living with the patient. Women account for 70 to 80 percent of the primary caregivers and range in age from the teens to the nineties. About one-third of the caregivers are entirely unassisted. They spend an average of about seventy hours a week at their task. If they do not work outside the home, they often spend as many as 100 hours a week at caregiving.

These people are trying to cope with their loved one's fear, loss of memory, incontinence, hiding or losing things, depression, stubbornness, repetition of insignificant events and details, and possibly sexual misconduct. Two-thirds of all caregivers say that their loved one cannot bathe, dress, or toilet without assistance. When you see them, most caregivers are weary, exhausted physically and emotionally. Ninety percent call it frustrating, draining, and painful. Three-fourths of them say they often feel depressed. Half feel that their marital relationship is threatened.

Many caregivers secretly (or not so secretly) feel abandoned by God—hearing nothing but silence from heaven. All too often they also feel abandoned by their faith community. Indeed, as I stated earlier, those who are forced by illness to stay at home for as long as a year are truly in danger of being abandoned. This belief was first based on observation and then confirmed by research (Justice, 1991).

Families of Alzheimer's disease need support—support that begins with compassionate messages of encouragement from the pulpit and extends to sympathetic conversations over coffee or at the bedside. After the ministering person has listened and listened, and listened, to the frustrations, anxieties, pain, helplessness, and hopelessness, the caregiver will be hoping for some good news. At the heart of the gospel is the good news that God wishes to save, not only from some torment beyond but from the torment of the here and now. Heaven is not truly silent when God's representative speaks confidently from his written word.

Force yourself sometimes to sit silently with the patient. On occasion, you also may need to do the same with members of the family. I personally believe that the ministry of silence is one of our most neglected ministries. Patients who are seriously ill or terribly weary typically do not experience the awkwardness of silence that so pervades our culture. Most of us require uninterrupted sound when we are with another person. When you minister to patients who are truly unable to communicate or you do not know their level of understanding, remember that people often have feelings they cannot put into words. Your presence may be understood even if your words are not. Your presence may speak of love. Your tender voice or your pleasant smile may reach the patient at an unknown level. These may also reassure of your compassion. Don't underestimate God. Remember that some of God's most important messages have been delivered by the most unlikely people. You may never know what our Lord is able to communicate through you to that "impossible" person *even when you are unaware of it.*

Indeed, you probably will never know this side of heaven what any visit has meant. When you decide to make your visit with the sick more than a social call, pray that God will help you to make it a ministry. Less than a week ago, I was introduced to a person who responded, "Oh! We've met before! You visited our family when Papa was so terribly sick. I want to thank you for what you meant to us at that time." I was embarrassed. I didn't remember. I had made that visit more than fifteen years ago. Those to whom you minister during difficult times will remember you long after you have forgotten them.

Chapter 9

Conclusion

"I was sick and you visited me," said our Lord Jesus. His listeners could not even remember ever having seen him sick. "When did we do that?" they asked. He replied, "Inasmuch as ye have done it unto one of the least of these my brethren, ye have done it unto me" (Matt. 25:34-40). I'm not sure I have ever understood all the implications of those words. I do understand that when we reach out to minister to someone who is ill, in some very real, concrete way we are serving Jesus, the Savior and King. Perhaps that is all we need to understand.

The word *visit* has a verb form. It is action. When we visit, we are doing something for our Lord while we are doing something for another person. We do not visit by accident. With each visit we give something of ourselves. We sacrifice time and energy that could have been used in any of a thousand different ways, many of which would be more pleasurable to ourselves. When we put love into action, our Lord heartily approves.

Until well into my adult years, when someone spoke of the judgment of God, I understood it as futuristic and being only negative. In essence, I was hearing a version of, "God's going to get you for that!" "That" could be any of a million wrongs that I might have done.

Then, one day I saw the judgment of God as a daily experience—on this side of eternity. *Every day is judgment day.* Yes, when you have not done as you should, listen carefully and you may hear a quiet voice somewhere deep within your soul telling you that you have sinned. Some student of psychology may tell us that the voice is only our own conscience. Although my psychological studies and counseling experiences are as thorough as those of many psychologists, I'm still convinced that a "still, small voice" often comes from beyond our own mind. When you have done that which you should have done, you also are likely to hear a quiet little voice somewhere deep within your soul saying, "Well done."

Jesus spoke a parable about a man who had entrusted talents of various sizes into the care of his servants before he went on a trip. Some put their talents to work, and in doing so the talents were multiplied. One buried his talent without use. When the master returned and asked for an accounting of the talents, he judged the caretakers on the basis of their behavior. He rewarded those who had multiplied the money entrusted to them, and he judged harshly the one who had buried his talent, having failed to use it.

However large or small you may see your "talent" for ministering to the sick, you are working to make it grow. Your having read this book is evidence of that fact. Seek God's help and put what you learn by study and experience into practice. As you do, listen and you just may hear, "I was sick and ye visited me. . . . As ye have done it unto the least of these my brothers, ye have done it unto me. . . . Well done, good and faithful servant" (Matt. 25:14-23).

Then, bow your head and say, "Thank You, Lord, for the privilege of having served."

References

Carnegie, Dale (1982). *How to Win Friends and Influence People.* New York: Pocket Books, Inc.

Glasser, Barney G. and Strauss, Anselm L. (1968). *Awareness of Dying.* Chicago: Aldine Publishing Co. (Although this is an old book, it is an excellent resource for anyone who wants to pursue this subject. During the final days of preparation of this manuscript, several copies were available at Amazon.com.)

Griffith, Jerry and Standberg, Twila (1982). *A Guide to Nursing Home Living.* Charleston, IL: Generations Publishing Co., p. 33ff. (Although more than twenty years old, this work offers suggestions that are appropriate for today's patients. It is out of print, but available on the Internet.)

Justice, William G. (1973). *Don't Sit on the Bed: A Handbook for Visiting the Sick.* Nashville, TN: Broadman Press.

Justice, William G. (1980). *Guilt and Forgiveness.* Grand Rapids, MI: Baker Book House, 1980. (This book is out of print, but sometimes available in used book stores and at Amazon.com and Barnesandnoble. com.)

Justice, William G. (1991). "A Survey Report of Nursing Home Ministry and Perceived Needs with Implications for Pastoral Care." *Journal of Religious Gerontology,* 8(2):101-110. (Although this research was completed several years ago, I have no reason to think it would reveal anything different if it had been conducted more recently. If you conduct a similar inquiry in your own region, I hope the results will be completely different. Two or three interviews will suffice.)

Justice, William G. (2004). *God in the Hands of Angry Sinners.* Bloomington, IL: Authorhouse.

Kübler-Ross, Elisabeth (1969). *On Death and Dying.* New York: Macmillan Co.

Lockerbie, Bruce D. (1998). *Dismissing God.* Grand Rapids, MI: Baker Book House, p. 141.

Serocki, Elena (2001). "Heaven Can Wait." *Reader's Digest,* May, p. 112.

Strohl, Linda (2001). "Why Doctors Now Believe Faith Heals: Because They're Finding Medical Evidence." *Reader's Digest,* May, pp. 108-115.

USDA (1999). USDA Release No. 0176.99. Author.

Index

THE HAWORTH PASTORAL PRESS®
Pastoral Care, Ministry, and Spirituality
Richard Dayringer, ThD
Senior Editor

BECOMING A FORGIVING PERSON: A PASTORAL PERSPECTIVE by Henry Close. "*Becoming A Forgiving Person* is a tender and compelling work that charts differing paths which lead to personal healing through the medium of forgiveness. Close's wisdom of psyche and soul come together in very practical ways through his myriad stories and illustrations." *Virginia Felder, MDiv, ThM, DMin, Licensed Professional Counselor, Licensed Marriage and Family Therapist, Private Practice, Dallas, TX*

A PASTORAL COUNSELOR'S MODEL FOR WELLNESS IN THE WORK-PLACE: PSYCHERGONOMICS by Robert L. Menz. "This text is a must-read for chaplains and pastoral counselors wishing to understand and apply holistic health care to troubled employees, whether they be nurses, physicians, other health care workers, or workers in other industries. This book is filled with practical ideas and tools to help clergy care for the physical, mental, and spiritual needs of employees at the workplace." *Harold G. Koenig, MD, Associate Professor of Psychiatry, Duke University Medical Center; Author,* Chronic Pain: Biomedical and Spiritual Approaches

A THEOLOGY OF PASTORAL PSYCHOTHERAPY: GOD'S PLAY IN SACRED SPACES by Brian W. Grant. "Brian Grant's book is a compassionate and sophisticated synthesis of theology and psychoanalysis. His wise, warm grasp binds a community of healers with the personal qualities, responsibilities, and burdens of the pastoral psychotherapist." *David E. Scharff, MD, Co-Director, International Institute of Object Relations Therapy*

LOSSES IN LATER LIFE: A NEW WAY OF WALKING WITH GOD, SECOND EDITION by R. Scott Sullender. "Continues to be a timely and helpful book. There is an empathetic tone throughout, even though the book is a bold challenge to grieve for the sake of growth and maturity and faithfulness. . . . An important book." *Herbert Anderson, PhD, Professor of Pastoral Theology, Catholic Theological Union, Chicago, Illinois*

CARING FOR PEOPLE FROM BIRTH TO DEATH edited by James E. Hightower Jr. "An expertly detailed account of the hopes and hazards folks experience at each stage of their lives. Your empathy will be deepened and your care of people will be highly informed." *Wayne E. Oates, PhD, Professor of Psychiatry Emeritus, School of Medicine, University of Louisville, Kentucky*

HIDDEN ADDICTIONS: A PASTORAL RESPONSE TO THE ABUSE OF LEGAL DRUGS by Bridget Clare McKeever. "This text is a must-read for physicians, pastors, nurses, and counselors. It should be required reading in every seminary and Clinical Pastoral Education program." *Martin C. Helldorfer, DMin, Vice President, Mission, Leadership Development and Corporate Culture, Catholic Health Initiatives—Eastern Region, Pennsylvania*

THE EIGHT MASKS OF MEN: A PRACTICAL GUIDE IN SPIRITUAL GROWTH FOR MEN OF THE CHRISTIAN FAITH by Frederick G. Grosse. "Thoroughly grounded in traditional Christian spirituality and thoughtfully aware of the needs of men in our culture. . . . Close attention could make men's groups once again a vital spiritual force in the church." *Eric O. Springsted, PhD, Chaplain and Professor of Philosophy and Religion, Illinois College, Jacksonville, Illinois*

THE HEART OF PASTORAL COUNSELING: HEALING THROUGH RELATION-SHIP, REVISED EDITION by Richard Dayringer. "Richard Dayringer's revised edition of *The Heart of Pastoral Counseling* is a book for every person's pastor and a pastor's every person." *Glen W. Davidson, Professor, New Mexico Highlands University, Las Vegas, New Mexico*

WHEN LIFE MEETS DEATH: STORIES OF DEATH AND DYING, TRUTH AND COURAGE by Thomas W. Shane. "A kaleidoscope of compassionate, artfully tendered pastoral encounters that evoke in the reader a full range of emotions." *The Rev. Dr. James M. Harper, III, Corporate Director of Clinical Pastoral Education, Health Midwest; Director of Pastoral Care, Baptist Medical Center and Research Medical Center, Kansas City Missouri*

A MEMOIR OF A PASTORAL COUNSELING PRACTICE by Robert L. Menz. "Challenges the reader's belief system. A humorous and abstract book that begs to be read again, and even again." *Richard Dayringer, ThD, Professor and Director, Program in Psychosocial Care, Department of Medical Humanities; Professor and Chief, Division of Behavioral Science, Department of Family and Community Medicine, Southern Illinois University School of Medicine*

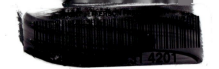